ADVENTURES OF A DISEASE DETECTIVE

Written by Mark E White
Designed by Zoe Z White

Published by Cone Shell Books

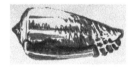

ABOUT THE AUTHOR

Mark White graduated from Michigan State University's Justin Morrel College magna cum laude in 1969, then the University of Michigan School of Medicine. He completed a residency there and an Infectious Diseases Fellowship at the Peter Bent Brigham Hospital (now Mass General Brigham).

Mark joined the Centers for Disease Control and Prevention's Epidemic Intelligence Serve and then spent six years as the bubonic plague epidemiologist for CDC. When his first wife left and took their children, Alex and Daniel, to the east coast, he followed and found a job as Hospital Epidemiologist at Booth Memorial Medical Center (now New York Presbyterian Queens). While investigating a head lice outbreak in the Respiratory Intensive Unit, he met and eventually married Felilia (Budsy) Mendoza, the beautiful head nurse.

In 1986, when the People Power revolution overthrew the corrupt Marcos government in Manila, Budsy and Mark joined the Philippine Department of Health to help set up a CDC-type epidemiology unit. Over seven years, they investigated Ebola virus, typhoid, cholera, malaria, and AIDS outbreaks, as well as mass poisonings with shellfish toxins and embalming fluid (formaldehyde). They were on the slopes of Mount Pinatubo when it erupted, lowering the global temperature by two degrees C for two years, and helped supervise the care of 140,000 evacuees. They endured six military coup attempts.

Budsy got breast cancer and had chemotherapy. They moved to Uganda, which was recovering from the effects of the dictatorships of Idi Amin and his successors. They investigated tropical diseases and narrowly escaped a plot to murder them.

They moved to Atlanta, where CDC appointed Mark Director of the Division of International Health. He helped create new training programs in China, India, Kenya, Central Asia, and Central America. A year after Budsy died, Mark married Shelly Ahmann, a breast surgeon. They are happily wed 23 years later. They adopted two beautiful sisters from Ethiopia, Leila and Zebedia.

Mark retired in 2012 and has been writing this memoir since.

ADVANCE PRAISE FOR ADVENTURES OF A DISEASE DETECTIVE

Look out, Dr. Fauci, here comes a disease detective who equals your expertise with medicine and people! This book is heartfelt, sexy, and adventuresome! Be sure to grab a snack before starting because you won't be able to put it down! —**Dr. Marti Loring, author of** *Intimate Behavior*

Intense true tales—and engaging personal tidbits—from the front lines of international medicine. White exhibits both a clever sense of humor and a graphic, descriptive flair for language." —**Kirkus Reviews**

Mark White is a real-life medical detective. This engaging book gives a personal and professional account of the trials, tribulations, successes, and failures of his varied undertakings around the world. An important and salutary read for any aspiring medical detective! —**Peter Smith, Professor of Tropical Epidemiology, London School of Hygiene & Tropical Medicine**

This narrative of epidemics and disasters faced and dealt with will engage you – particularly if you like mystery diseases and their solutions…. Half the characters were persons that I knew. Mark's prose brings them to life with humor. It was better than reading a novel. —**Manuel M. Dayrit, former Secretary of the Philippine Department of Health and Director of Human Resources of the World Health Organization**, was dean of the Ateneo School of Medicine and Public Health. Now he is an emeritus professor

For readers, the exotic locations and insights allow us to see the world through a microscope and observe doctors stopping the spread of disease. The book places readers in a new wider world of compassion and understanding. And with all the drama, there is always room for humor. It sustains us all.

—**Carol Lee Lorenzo, author of Nervous Dancer** (winner of Flannery O'Connor Award.) Her most recent novel is *Sleeping in Public*

ISBN 979-8-9878076-0-6

This book was written by Mark Edward White in his private capacity. No
official support or endorsement by the US government, World Health
Organization, Rockefeller Foundation, the Philippine, Ugandan, or other
governments is intended or should be inferred.

This book is dedicated to my mom, Betty White, and my dad, Elmer White. Mom wanted me to be a diplomat, and dad wanted me to be a writer. He typed my childish stories and mimeographed pamphlets of them for his friends. Mom saved every story I wrote. I wish they were alive to see this book.

My life has been beautiful because of my wives, Budsy and Shelly, and my children, Alex, Daniel, Leila, and ZuZu; my grandkids, Ry and Casey; and my siblings, Marty Jo Campbell and Thomas Eliot White.

These stories are especially dedicated to Conchy Roces, Conky Lim-Quizon, my other students, and their students.

Alan Barnes, Mario Taguiwalo, Dioniso Herrera, Tim Dean, Tom Keever, Hal Margolis, and Alfredo RA Bengzon made the world a better place before they died. I miss them.

My songs will not come to an end.
My stories will not come to an end.
I, the singer, raise them up.
They are scattered.
They are bestowed.

—*Ancient Mayan Hymn, revised by John Ciardi*

CONTENTS

INTRODUCTION

For the best part of my career, I was a disease detective helping developing countries stop and prevent epidemics the way we did at the Centers for Disease Control and Prevention (CDC). My wife, Budsy, and I worked in ministries of health around the world to build epidemiology programs and train disease detectives.

COVID-19 and monkeypox (mpox to the politically correct) arrived after the time this book covers, but the lessons still apply. Politicians took over CDC's technical reporting early in the COVID-19 pandemic and suppressed truthful reports. This wasn't CDC's fault, and the present negative press about the agency is undeserved and unfair.

These stories are as true as I could make them. Whenever possible, I sent chapters to the people who appeared in them so they could check the facts. The results were sometimes painful, but I made the changes. At least one person reviewed nearly every chapter. Of course, nobody can remember long-ago conversations, so I made them up.

These are not tall tales. The appendix at the end of this book contains a bibliography of representative scientific papers my colleagues and I wrote about our shared adventures.

I hope you have as much fun reading these stories as I had living them.

—Mark White, Atlanta, 2022

CHAPTER 1
FLUSHING NEW YORK IS A GOOD IDEA

hapter 1: Flushing New York is a Good Idea

In 1987, I was the bubonic plague specialist for the Centers for Disease Control (CDC) when my first wife, tired of my traveling, left me. She took the kids and moved to Boston, where she became an eminent neuropsychologist. To be closer to them, I found a job as a hospital epidemiologist at Booth Memorial Medical Center in Queens, New York.

I moved in with my best friend, Tom Dale Keever, a Shakespearean actor, who lived in a tiny efficiency apartment in Manhattan's Hell's Kitchen neighborhood, at Forty-Fifth Street and Tenth Avenue, in a four-story walk-up above a salsa record studio. It was incredibly close to the big theaters, which was great for him but of limited utility for me.

When you walked out the door of his building, you could look down the street and see the hulking World War II aircraft carrier, the *Intrepid*, which is now a museum. Tom called it "my neighborhood aircraft carrier."

Keever was a bit eccentric. He mostly ate tuna, and his mantle sported a giant pyramid of empty tuna cans. The crowning glory of the apartment was the bathtub, which stood in the middle of the room, topped with a door. This served as the table. A tiny kitchen and bathroom completed the amenities.

Tom once played Macbeth in an off-off-Broadway production. "The *New York Times* reviewed the show," he told me. "They said it sucked, and it was all my fault. Fuck 'em if they can't take a joke."

Words to live by.

Back in those days, New York was tough. One day I walked into the lobby of Tom's building and found two junkies shooting up. I fled up the stairs and got Tom. When we looked down the stairs, the junkies hid their works under the linoleum.

Tom said, "We better call the police. Once, I heard a rape going on behind the building. Four police cars were here in five minutes. The station is just up the road."

Nobody came.

Indignant, we decided to confront the police. When we reached the foot of the stairs, I found the junkies' works and snatched them up. Evidence.

The junkies were dozing on the sidewalk as we walked out the door. Now we were committed to involving the cops.

We headed down to the station and explained our problem. "Here's proof," I said and smacked the works on the sergeant's desk.

He stared. Finally, he said, "I can't decide whether I should book you for possession of narcotics or put this in the lost and found."

Tom said, "What?"

Suddenly, a lieutenant appeared behind us and led us to an interrogation room. He was a trim fellow with a little mustache. "Here's the deal. If I arrest these guys, they'll be out of jail the same day. Think of the junkies as an infestation of vermin. There's only one way to get them out of the building. If you swear you saw them buying and selling dope, we can put them out of circulation for a couple of years."

Tom and I said, "We didn't see them sell drugs."

The lieutenant said, "I can't hear you. What's that again?" He seemed disappointed. "Let me know if you see a sale." Then he released us.

Back at the apartment building, the junkies were gone. We were afraid they'd be back with knives, but we never saw them again.

Another tale from the naked city.

Tom introduced me to a sweet and lovely Columbia graduate student named Jessica. She had luxuriant, wavy brown hair and soulful brown eyes. I soon moved in with her on 113th Street. When you walked out the front door and turned left, you faced the mighty facade of the Cathedral of Saint John the Divine. Manhattan is amazing.

Jessica and I lived the high life in "the city," as opposed to the "bridge and tunnel" peasants who dwelled in the darkness of the outer boroughs. Of course, Queens was, and is, one of these boroughs. My hospital was in Flushing, Queens. You have no idea how many people sent Christmas cards saying, "Flushing New York is a good idea."

Driving to Booth was easy because I was going against the traffic. I sometimes had to rush to the hospital in the middle of the night to handle emergencies. The most direct route was to go up to 125th Street, then head to the Triborough Bridge.

Once, I had to drive to Queens for an emergency at 2:00 a.m. I had an almost-new Ford Escort with front-wheel drive. I sailed through green lights crossing Harlem until Second Avenue when a guy in a big car ran the red light and smashed into my side. He backed up, untangled his vehicle from mine with a sickening screeching of metal, then disappeared uptown.

I climbed out and walked shakily to a gas station to call AAA. Life was more complicated before we all got cell phones.

"We don't make pickups there at night," a nasal, nasty voice informed me.

"Do you make pickups in the day?" I tried to sound sarcastic to cover the fear shooting up into my chest.

"Sometimes," he said, then hung up.

I couldn't get a taxi either.

I needed to think. I inspected the car to see whether I could bend something to get it rolling again. No luck.

Voices came from close behind me. "Hey, man, did you see the license plate on the car that hit you?"

I spun. "No."

"Well, we did."

"Thanks. Tell me, and I'll memorize it."

"It don't work that way. You pay us, and we tell you."

There were at least six of them, young kids wearing black leather jackets. They nudged closer, and I backed up. Somehow they got me into a dark place behind a dumpster. At least the sanitation people would find my body.

"You got fifty dollars? Show us your wallet."

A tiny ray of hope. They wanted to negotiate. "Look, guys, the number won't be any good. It's probably a stolen car."

"Yeah, lots of those 'round here, 'specially at night. So what will you pay us?"

"How about a dollar."

"Man, man. You're not respect'n us," the leader whined. They began pushing me back against the dumpster.

I looked in my wallet. "How about five?"

"Deal."

After the kids left, I moved to the center of 125th Street. I felt safer there. Nobody came. Then a tall black guy walked out of the gas station holding two cups of coffee.

"Have a cup. Looks like you had an accident."

"Yes," I replied. "I can't get the car towed, and no taxi will pick me up."

"That sucks. Look, my uncle has a garage right around the

corner. I'll help you push it there, and then you can pick it up tomorrow."

"Wow. Thanks."

We managed to push it a couple of hundred feet to a closed garage door. My new friend knocked on the door and said something. It opened. Inside were blazing lights, a vision of hell. People were cutting up cars with welding torches, taking off license plates, stacking doors against walls, and yanking out engines.

"Holy shit!"

"Yeah, it's a chop shop."

"How do I know your uncle's not going to chop mine up?"

"My family decides what to chop, and with all due respect, there's not much market for Ford Escorts."

"I hadn't thought of that."

"Come on. I'll borrow a car and drive you home."

When we arrived, he leaned across the seat. "This is gonna cost you a hundred bucks, buddy."

"I don't have that much."

"Look. When I go to court, I have to pay hundreds of dollars to lawyers. They know the rules, got the contacts, know what I mean?"

"Yes."

"Think of me as a lawyer of the streets. I'll extend you credit till I pick you up in the morning."

"How can you be sure I'll pay?"

"I know where you live, man. Besides, I can sell the battery and tires of the Escort for more than that. I'm doing you a favor."

"Yes, you are," I replied.

I walked into our apartment, called the doctors at Booth who needed help, and talked them through their problems. Then I fell into the blackness of the sort of deep sleep soldiers fall into after being scared out of their wits in battle. In the morning, my "lawyer" picked me up and took me to the chop shop. My car was parked neatly out front.

"The mechanics tried to fix it for you, but we don't do transaxles. Here's a phone number to call a tow truck. Help me push it out into the street."

I paid him the hundred bucks plus a ten-dollar tip and took a taxi to work.

CHAPTER 2
IN CASE OF EMERGENCY

On my first day at Booth Memorial Medical Center, I pushed through the big glass front doors and came face-to-face with a tallish woman, black hair flowing down the back of her long white coat. She wore a crimson sweater. "Hi, I'm Barbara Russo, the Hospital Nurse Epidemiologist. Welcome. We have an emergency."

I opened my mouth to speak, but Barbara said, "This is Peggy, my assistant." Barbara smiled at a willowy strawberry blonde with a healthy pink complexion and pale blue eyes. She slipped around behind me and helped my arms into the sleeves of a white coat. "The medical department secretary estimated your size."

They led me double-time to the central elevator banks. "It's in the Respiratory Intensive Care Unit on the eighth floor," Barbara said through tight lips.

"What's the matter?"

"It's too horrible. I can't bring myself to tell you in a public place."

"I can't face a horror without a cup of coffee."

Barbara and Peggy shared a glance and led me into the coffee shop. Barbara told the cashier, "He's in a hurry. Get him a coffee with milk."

"I said, "Make the coffee black and add a bagel with cream cheese. Ms. Russo, I'm feeling hypoglycemic."

Peggy led me to a table. Barbara said, "No need to sit down. I'll get the coffee to go."

"And the bagel. That, too."

Barbara shook her head, paid, looked thoughtful, and said, "Toast the bagel."

A flush of gratefulness swept through me. Barbara carried the coffee over and handed it to me. "They'll send the bagel up when it's done." I could feel Peggy's breath on my head as she stood behind me.

"Ms. Russo…"

"Call me Barbara."

"Barbara, the bagel will take about three minutes, and one's already passed."

Barbara sat down and leaned close to my face. "It's the head nurse in the Respiratory ICU. It's terrible what she's done."

Clearly, she would say no more. We sat silently until the cashier said, "One toasted bagel up."

I hurried up and took a bite on the way back to our table.

Peggy snatched the bagel, rewrapped it, and shoved it into my coat pocket.

Five minutes later, they marched me into the humming, beeping sunlight of the Respiratory ICU. There are always big glass windows in these places. Most patients are in comas with their eyes taped shut to keep them from drying out. I'm sure the nurses like the windows. It softens the pain of spending days among sick and dying people as they treat and nurture them.

The unit was one huge room. Beds stood against the walls, and a nursing station was directly across from the doors. Doctors and nurses made rounds in little groups, murmuring to each other.

As I took this all in, a small woman in a cute frilly nurse's cap and a white minidress charged at us like a heat-seeking missile. She was maybe four feet ten in black heels. She pinned me with flashing dark eyes. Her little dress set off her smooth, brown skin.

She'd been expecting us.

"I'm Miss Mendoza, the head nurse."

Barbara extended her arm and pointed like an ancient prophet at an old lady sitting in a chair in a corner. A respirator tube extended from her mouth. Air hissed into the machine, then blew it back out a few seconds later. She wore a colorful handkerchief on her head like an old gypsy. She moved her hands as if sewing invisible cloth.

Miss Mendoza led us to her. "Meet Mrs. Feinstein." The old lady's head popped up, looking at us happily. "Her family put her in one of our fine local nursing homes, where she got pneumonia. They transferred her to us. We stabilized her on the ventilator when I noticed a spot on her nurse's white sweater. When I saw it move, I knew it was a bug, a head louse. I saw lots of them in the Philippines."

So she was from the Philippines. That explained her brown complexion and trim, strong legs. Barbara later told me the nursing department had ordered her to wear longer dresses. She ignored them, proof of Miss Mendoza's lawless character.

"I see," I said. I looked at Barbara. "Is this the emergency?" Peggy looked out the window. I couldn't tell whether she was concealing a smile.

Miss Mendoza looked me directly in the eyes as she recited, "Today is the first of July, and I noticed the lice at about 3:00 a.m. I notified the resident on call, but it was his first day, and he didn't know what to do. He said to call you in the morning, so I told my nurse to take off her sweater, comb out her hair and go home. None of my other nurses wanted to care for Mrs. Feinstein for fear of infecting their families. I've been up more than twenty-four hours, and I need to rest. I had to do something."

She peered at me like an angry tropical bird. "I couldn't tolerate head lice in my unit, so I did what we did in the Philippines—I had the hospital barber shave her head."

This is a highly effective remedy. Head lice can't stick to bare skin because they have only two pinchers that look like lobster claws. They cling to individual hair shafts and swing from hair to hair the way Tarzan swings through the forest.

"No hair, no lice. That should do the trick," I said. "So what's the problem?"

"My staff won't come near her, and I'm afraid I won't be able to staff the night shift. They all have kids."

"We can be sure to kill all lice by washing her hair with Kwell shampoo. It's highly effective against head lice. You don't even need a prescription. You can get it at any pharmacy."

Miss Mendoza cleared her throat. "I called the pharmacy to ask if they had anything for head lice. They told me about Kwell, but they don't stock it. They said a family member could pick it up from any drugstore nearby."

A trim professional-looking woman in a long white coat strode into the unit. Her hair was pulled back in a severe bun, and her high heels clicked on the linoleum. "I'm Mrs. Pappas. I'm the hospital barber."

Peggy said, "I paged her to tell her side of the story."

Mrs. Pappas glared. "In my twenty-five years of service here, nobody has ever taken a patient's clippings without their consent."

Miss Mendoza smiled. "Did you ask her?"

"Of course not; she's not of sound mind. The hair belongs to her family. After I shaved the old lady, you snatched up the bag of hair and destroyed her private property." She cast her eyes around our little group. "Miss Mendoza threw the hair into the incinerator. Of course, I reported her to the administration. She violated the rules."

"As you can see, the problem," Barbara said icily, "is that Miss Mendoza threw away hair that didn't belong to her. Now the hospital is liable if there's a lawsuit."

"Who'd want a bag full of head lice?" I asked.

Peggy was staring out the window again.

Mrs. Feinstein looked up at us, happily stitching her imaginary cloth. She was alone in the world, cared for by strangers, facing life by herself for her last years through her dementia. All in all, she did a good job.

Still, the situation was funny. I suppressed a smile. "I think we've got it under control for now. I'll write a note in the chart."

Barbara smiled with thin lips. "Saying what?"

"If the nursing staff had kept the bag of head lice in the unit, it would be an infectious hazard to the staff and visitors. I'll be happy to talk to the administrators."

Barbara's eyes widened with shock. "What about Miss Mendoza's behavior toward the barber? Barbers are professionals like us—and she was right about the regulations."

"It sounds like Miss Mendoza needs to go home and rest," I said.

The barber turned and marched away, followed by the nurse epidemiologists. Mrs. Feinstein and I watched Miss Mendoza walk briskly away. Her little white minidress glowed in the golden morning sun. I noticed a plaque on the wall behind the desk that said, IN EMERGENCY, BREAK GLASS. A little bottle of Lourdes Water and a wooden hammer were glued next to it.

Miss Mendoza turned to face me. "Call me Budsy," she said.

CHAPTER 3
CAUGHT BETWEEN TWO WOLVES

T hose first days in Booth were often sad and painful. Once, Joe invited Alice Trillin to give Grand Rounds on an essay she'd written in the New England Journal of Medicine about her soon-to-be fatal lung cancer. She was Calvin Trillin's wife and an author in her own right.

Fear and grief swept over me when she stepped up to the microphone. She looked so much like Bobbie. Ms. Trillin stood a few feet away from me as I listened to her mourning her lost life and love.

About halfway through her talk, I lurched to my feet and charged across the hall into Barbara Russo's office. She grabbed me into a tight hug, and I flooded her sweater with tears. We never talked about it later.

Tides of immigrants came to Queens. Flushing adsorbed them in waves, starting with the Dutch, English, then Irish, Greeks, and Italians, then Asians. Barbara was Italian, of course, and her sidekick, the Irish Peggy, was married to a Czech. Budsy was part of a vast influx of Asians that followed. They were not the huddled masses types but ambitious middle-class strivers. Years later, my next-door neighbor sold his house to a Hong Kong Chinese woman.

He said, "I was going to ask for more, but then she opened a little suitcase full of hundred-dollar bills."

A couple of years later, I met Mrs. Chen, a Chinese lady from Hong Kong. She'd developed the terrible immune disease systemic lupus erythematosus (SLE). Your immune system is designed to destroy invading threats by dissolving invaders with acid and harsh enzymes. If your white cells mistake your own tissues for enemies, they tear into every organ in your body and dissolve them. That's what happened to Mrs. Chen. You can die quickly. In English, Systemic Lupus Erythematosus means "the red wolf."

Her doctor put her on high-dose steroids to block the immune system. It seemed to work at first, but then she developed wracking fevers and seizures, and he called me.

When I entered her room, Mrs. Chen lay in her bed, thin and wan, covered with rashes. She was pushing a man away with a skinny arm.

"I'm her husband," he said. "I'm very worried about her."

She was shivering, a sign her temperature was going up. I said, "She is very sick. Please let me examine her."

He bowed like a waiter inviting you to sit down at a white-clothed table.

"I think it will be better if I examine her alone."

He left. Mrs. Chen looked up from her bed, eyes dull. Her skin was dry and slack, her muscles lax and rubbery. She smelled like skin lotion, rubbing alcohol, and unbrushed teeth. "My neck's stiff," she said.

I tried to bend her neck. It was so stiff I picked her up like a wooden plank. This is a sign of meningitis, inflammation around the brain.

She gasped.

"I'm sorry," I said.

Through gritted teeth, she said, "Please warn me if you do this again."

"I will. Sorry, Mrs. Chen."

She tensed and looked up at me, and took a deep breath.

Had her doctor known a little epidemiology, he'd have realized Asians had high rates of tuberculosis. TB is an unusual disease. Your body fights germs by attacking them with antibodies. Your white cells eat the bacteria and dissolve them. TB germs protect themselves by secreting a waxy cover that keeps antibodies and white blood cells from sticking to them. Plan B for the immune system is to wall them off with calcium and scar tissue to trap the bacteria. These lumps are called tubercles. They can get large and are distinctive on chest X-Rays. I have a few on my lungs, left over from exposure during my internship.

Unfortunately, the germs survive inside the tubercles. They can happily live inside for the rest of your life, waiting to break out if your immune system weakens. Eventually, everybody's immune system weakens from another disease or old age. The bacteria pour out into the bloodstream and attack every part of your body. The high doses of steroids her doctor put her on profoundly suppressed her immune system. She was a set up to die from TB.

Before I saw her X-rays, I knew that she almost certainly had miliary TB. A dreadful disease, it used to be called galloping consumption.

In the 1800s, pathologists did autopsies and found little hard abscesses all through the bodies, reminding them of tiny millet seeds. That's why it's called miliary. Imagine how dedicated and curious these men were. They knew they took the risk of getting what they called 'corpse fever.' Dissection was against the law, so these heroes often had to work in secret, frequently on smelly old corpses dug up from cemeteries.

In the nineteenth century, TB was called the white plague. In the Middle Ages, TB frequently affected the skin, causing lupus vulgaris, the "common wolf." Don't let anyone tell you it was great to live back when knighthood was in flower. TB was flowering, too.

Poor Mrs. Chen was being torn apart by the two wolves. She lay listlessly, looking up at me, too tired to talk. I started her on high-dose anti-TB drugs and admitted her to the intensive care unit. It was touch and go. The steroids were helping the TB spread, but cutting them would allow her lupus erythematosus back.

To justify cutting back on the steroids and treating her TB, I needed to see it on a biopsy. Taking a piece of her lung might kill her, but she had a swollen liver, and we could biopsy that. It was midnight, but I called my favorite surgeon, Jim Turner. He was the last of the heroic surgeons who stayed up all night, holding people's arteries together as they sprayed showers of blood. I always thought of him as the last survivor of the age of Iron Men and Wooden Heads. As an internist, I always put an article on the charts so residents could learn about the disease. Jim was the only surgeon who put journal articles under my door. I was vexed because it was my job to put articles under his door. That meant I had to look up two more articles.

I called him, and he came in at three a.m. and did the biopsy. At four, he called and woke me up. "She did well in surgery, sick as she was."

"No need to wake me up."

"Fuck you," he laughed.

I could hardly complain.

That morning the biopsy came back positive for TB. I could cut the steroids way back and start treating her for TB.

Eventually, she made it through and returned to her bed on the nursing floor. Since her recovery, she was quiet and ignored doctors when they tried to speak to her. I thought she might have brain damage or maybe an ICU psychosis. She'd more than earned some post-traumatic shock.

One morning I came in to make rounds. She looked up. "I don't want to see my husband. Can you keep him out of my room?"

"I'll talk to the head nurse. Is there something wrong?"

She looked up, peering into my eyes. "I'm divorcing him. When I got sick, he found my keys, and he's been digging through the apartment looking for money. He's a gambler. He's lost most of my money already. I curse the day I met him."

"Why are you asking me to keep him out? Didn't you see your other doctors earlier this morning?"

She said something like, "The other doctors are just Thais." She pointed to my neck. Eventually, I realized she only saw the other doctors' ties because she couldn't see the top of her visual field. I'm short, so she saw my face.

When tuberculosis attacks the brain, thick pus forms around the protective layer outside the brain, the dura mater. It means "hard mother" in Latin. The pus sinks down below the brain and pushes up on the optic nerves connecting your eyes to your brain. She could only see the top half of what she saw in front of her.

Mrs. Chen was a great save. Every single one of her doctors, nurses, and others was essential to saving her life.

Apparently, she managed to keep money away from her no-good, soon-to-be ex-husband because she paid my bill in full—in new hundred-dollar bills.

CHAPTER 4
THE 4-H CLUB

A fter the head lice fiasco, I said, "Mrs. Russo, it's my first day, and I need to see Dr. Dwek, head of the Internal Medicine Department."

Barbara took my arm. "No. First, we're meeting the Director of Nursing." I consider New York the world capital of rudeness. Mrs. Russo was a New Yorker in spades.

"Mrs. Russo, I need to see Dr. Dwek first."

"I moved your appointment by a half hour. We'll take you there as soon as we're done. Stop calling me Mrs. Russo. It's Barbara."

"Right." I sighed.

The Director of Nursing emphasized that she was eager to work with me—as long as I understood that Barbara and Peggy worked for her, not me.

Finally, they delivered me to Internal Medicine. Dr. Dwek looked up from his desk and raised his glasses to his forehead. "Welcome aboard, Mark. Tomorrow, we have Grand Rounds, and I've asked all the staff and residents to be sure to attend. I'll introduce you to the staff and residents then. You'll make the main presentation. We all want to hear what you have to offer, so talk about an interesting topic. See you then."

I was up most of the night drafting outline after outline

and thinking of amusing and enlightening anecdotes. After a few beers, I went to bed and tried to sleep.

At 7:00 a.m., my beeper went off. My first page! It was Barbara. "Good morning, champ. I hear you're presenting at Grand Rounds at nine."

"Is there anything you don't hear?"

"Not for very long. You'll thank me for it. Stop by my office at eight-thirty, and I'll show you where it is."

Barbara led me to the vast auditorium with two cups of coffee and a bagel in hand. The rows were stepped up steeply.

As I stood at the podium to begin my speech, there must have been over two hundred people in the audience. I told them stories about epidemics and rare infections, laced with jokes to cover my fear. I was in a bit of a haze, but there must have been some laughs because a resident came up to me afterward and said I could do stand-up.

Unfortunately, all was not funny. Two weeks before I moved to New York, I learned I'd failed the Internal Medicine qualifying exam. This was a big problem because Infectious Diseases is a subspecialty of Internal Medicine, so I had to pass both boards. I could still start at Booth, but in the eyes of the state, I was a general practitioner.

When I took the exam in Boston, my wife had just left me. I hoped to do better now that things were calmer. I took a review course, and a few weeks later, drove out to a test center on Long Island. I walked into an immense room and saw the first row was full of intense and nervous guys with bright Tensor desk lamps and rows of sharp No. 2 pencils on their desks. They had to sit in the front row to plug in the lights.

I was not the lone soul taking the test a second time.

This time, I passed.

I took a refresher course for the ID boards, too. I studied so hard that I could draw most antibiotics' structures and explain how they worked. I knew which sugars each common germ liked to eat and what parts of the body they infected.

As it turned out, I didn't need to know any of this. Most of the test was about tropical medicine—my forte. I passed with flying colors. The only question I couldn't answer was, "A fifteen-year-old Thai boy eats a lunch of raw water chestnuts and then flies to your city and consults you about severe epigastric (upper abdominal) pain. What is the most likely diagnosis?"

Years later, a smart Filipina microbiology technician told me the answer was *Fasciola hepatica*. It's an appalling flat-worm that spends part of its life in water chestnuts and the rest in your liver. It's about an inch long and grows in the bile ducts of your liver, chewing up tissue. It causes great pain, jaundice, high fevers, and sometimes death. It could be worse if you get the even larger *Fasciola gigantia*.

Passing boards is not enough. The science of medicine changes continuously. Important new papers are published every week, so you must keep up to give your patients the benefits of the latest discoveries. The best way to do this is by going to City Rounds where Infectious Diseases doctors from around the city meet and discuss hard cases for discussion. We often disagreed on diagnoses, and we'd tease and chal-lenge each other. If we disagreed, each of us would bring copies of articles, and we'd face off like cowboys at a gunfight.

New York City has superb rounds. I was once stumped by a man with pneumonia that turned out to be caused by fusar-ium, a fungus that causes diseases in grass and other plants. The poor guy developed a tumor that suppressed his immune system. He liked to garden and mow his lawn. His doctors started him on potent antibiotics to protect him from infec-tions, which killed all the bacteria and cleared the way for the grass fungus to get him. It's an infection that affects people with diminished immune systems, but I never guessed fusarium wilt. Who'd like that on his tombstone?

When it came time for me to present, I chose a chemist named Mr. Donegan, who specialized in making candy flavors. He had a herpes virus infection. The ancient Greek doctors first recorded herpes in wrestlers. When one wrestler had cold sores (caused by the herpes virus), he would drag his mouth across his opponent's skin. Painful, itchy vesicles (like you get in chickenpox) appeared and seemed to creep across the skin. Herpes in Greek means "I creep."

Poor Mr. Donegan had a cold sore that spread from the corner of his mouth across his cheek and consumed part of his ear. You could see his teeth and gums, like a skull. He had another sore that chewed up so much of his bottom that his anus looked like a little plateau on a bloody desert. He was in agony. We gave him lots of morphine, but it barely touched his pain. Surgeons tried cutting away the infected tissue, but that spread the damage faster. You usually see infections like this in patients who have suppressed immune systems. He wasn't on drugs that caused this, and I couldn't find signs of a tumor that might decrease his immune response.

A few months later, when it was my turn to present at city rounds, Mr. Donegan was my star patient. Doctors from Manhattan said he had Gay-Related Immune Deficiency (GRIDS), a new disease they'd started seeing a month ago. I went back and asked Mr. Donegan if he was gay. He denied it vehemently. As word spread, dozens of doctors asked him the same question from every angle, trying to trick him. It was the last straw. He began telling us he wanted to die in peace. It was a blessing that the disease soon spread far enough to kill him. Later, I learned he was infected by a blood transfusion.

I soon met my first gay patient with GRIDS, an airplane steward. He obviously wouldn't live long. I advised him to give his money to friends and family to avoid huge medical bills. The wan little man couldn't rise from lying down without help. He looked up at me. "I'm honest, and I will always be honest. You people have given me a few more days and relieved my pain."

He died with dignity. I hope I do as well.

Hospitals in California were reporting GRIDS, too. They found it among injecting drug users, hemophiliacs, and gays. They named it "Acquired Immunodeficiency Syndrome" (AIDS). The name stuck because the diseases affects people like Mr. Donegan in addition to gays. We remembered the risk factors as the 4-H Club: hemophiliacs, heroin abusers, homosexual men, and Haitians. The common factor was that these groups had many blood-borne diseases like hepatitis and syphilis.

Caring for AIDS patients slammed me emotionally. You expect old people to die. It's their time. AIDS patients were middle class, like me— and they were younger. I never got used to it.

My next AIDS patient was an IV drug user, a young woman named Cheryl Acocella. She came in with an unusual pneumonia caused by *Pneumocystis carinii*, a tiny parasite that usually lives in our lungs and minds its own business. If you have a damaged immune system, *Pneumocystis* may attack and cause terrible pneumonia. Fortunately for Cheryl, I could treat it with a pill used to treat urinary tract infections. One afternoon, I came into her room to find a psychiatry resident interviewing her with a video camera. She preened and ran her fingers through her hair. "Heroin is so great. It's worth getting AIDS. I'd do it all again."

She had a cringing nastiness that reminded me of the rats I trapped in New Mexico when I investigated bubonic plague cases. Cheryl and her overbearing mother demanded morphine to keep her from withdrawing from her addiction while in the hospital. When I discharged her, I referred her to a methadone clinic. We were all glad to part.

Her mother got hold of my home phone number a week later and woke me up at 3:00 a.m. Her daughter needed a fix right now. She ordered me to call in a prescription for morphine. "Mrs. Acocella, you can't call in prescriptions for narcotics. She'll have to go to the Emergency Room if she wants drugs."

"Fine. Meet us there in twenty minutes."

"No, the doctors there will evaluate her and decide what to give her. She can see me at my office in the morning. I won't write her a prescription for anything but drugs for her infections. I'll refer her to an addiction specialist."

She hung up.

A week later, Barbara Russo called me. "The state sent an investigator because a patient says you abused them. You can meet them in my office."

Barbara introduced me to the inspector, a large black woman in a long white coat. Her eyes protruded slightly, and she looked me up and down like I was an overflowing garbage can.

"Here's the letter," Barbara said. "It's from Mrs. Acocella. She says you denied her daughter essential medicines."

Amazingly, Mrs. Acocella described our phone call accurately. I looked up at the investigator. I was beginning to think of her as the hanging judge. "Do you see anything wrong with what I did?"

"No," the investigator said. I thought I caught a tinge of regret in her voice. "But we have to check each case in person." Then she left.

Barbara said, "I saved a copy of the letter for you."

I ripped it up and threw it in the wastebasket.

A few months later, Cheryl and her mother were back. This time, she had an overwhelming infection with a fungus, and it nearly killed her. After a month, she was well enough to be weaned off the ventilator. She asked for the psychiatry resident. This time, Cheryl said the horrors of her infections far outweighed the pleasures of heroin.

She didn't last long after that.

Haitians have a high rate of blood-borne infections, and AIDS cut a swath through them. A Haitian nurse asked me to see her sister, a midwife who had worked for several years in the Congo. There's a lot of blood during deliveries, and the virus must have infected her then. Now she had florid AIDS. I could do nothing except treat the curable infections and control her pain. Considering that she had an incurable disease and would soon die, there was no use putting her in the Intensive Care Unit. I admitted her to a private room. I saw her at about 11:00 p.m. when a nurse intercepted me. "Her whole family's in there. They're lighting candles and praying. I don't mind letting them stay after visiting hours, but it's against hospital rules to burn candles."

"I'll write a note taking responsibility for the candles."

She smiled wearily. "Thanks."

The midwife died that night.

We knew how to protect people against infection within weeks of seeing the first cases. What the 4-H club members had in common was a high rate of hepatitis B and syphilis, which are transmitted through blood and sex. AIDS behaved the same way, so it was clear that AIDS was also transmitted through blood and sex. Someone once defined epidemiology as "common sense applied to medicine." Knowing how AIDS was transmitted from person to person allowed us to stop it from spreading before we knew that a virus caused it.

When people think of scientists finding new diseases, they imagine immaculate, white-clad researchers holding vials of colored liquids in shiny labs. More often, it's scruffy characters doing detective work by grubbing around sewers and poking their noses into people's private business. People like me. Occasionally, I sent samples to high-security labs, where people wearing space suits grow and characterize dangerous viruses like Ebola. I have nothing against labs. I always wanted to work in a high-level lab but never got the chance.

It took two years for virologists to identify the virus that causes AIDS, the Human Immunodeficiency Virus (HIV). It infects the white blood cells that are the first responders to new infections. By the time your body makes antibodies, HIV is safe inside many cells, where antibodies can't reach them, so the infection continues. Usually, it takes months or years before people get sick with the disease. All this time, their blood is infectious—long before anybody knows they're sick. Tuberculosis and other chronic infectious diseases use similar strategies.

While antibodies can't protect you from HIV, they provide a marker for infection. We now have effective antiviral drugs that give AIDS patients decades of normal life. It's a triumph of science that this was worked out a couple of years after the disease emerged. It shows what an international effort can do when a new pandemic appears, as happened with the COVID-19 pandemic.

CDC and New York City quickly crafted guidelines on the best ways to keep health workers safe from HIV. Barbara and I spread the good news in meetings with all the major departments. Nobody believed us. Many doubters insisted we do the part of their job that worried them. People said pretty much the same things: "I worry that if I die, there'll be no one to support the wife and kids;" "With a disease this terrible, even the tiniest risk of infection is unacceptable;" and so on.

So for weeks, Barbara, Peggy, and I did the risky work needed to treat these patients to show that we weren't afraid. We were nervous, of course, but we knew the guidelines would work. We handed out meal trays to all the AIDS patients and carried the dirty dishes back to the kitchen. We bandaged wounds, tested blood in the lab, and helped with surgery, where the risk was minute because everybody was gowned and gloved. The only danger is if you cut through a glove and get some blood inside. The most memorable time was when I helped a proctologist biopsy a tumor in an AIDS patient's bowel. It involved spraying and sucking back contaminated fluids to find tumors to cut out. It was bloody work, but the proctologist easily stopped the bleeding with a hot wire. Because the procedures were so messy, everyone was masked, gowned, and double-gloved. We all wore goggles. Every flat surface in the operating room was covered with disposable paper drapes. Between each case, they rewashed and rewrapped everyone and everything.

I've always admired proctologists and rectal surgeons. People look down on such work—until they get a thrombosed hemorrhoid or bright red rectal bleeding.

CHAPTER 5
DON'T DRINK THE GREEN WATER

'd worked at Booth for a couple of years when Barbara called me at home at 5:00 a.m. "Better get in right now. There's something terribly wrong with the water. Nobody can drink it."

"I'll make a cup of coffee and come right in."

"We need you now. I'll give you a cup of coffee later. It's urgent. It's bad." She hung up.

I lived in a ratty apartment building a half block from the hospital, so I was there in fifteen minutes. On the way to Barbara's office, I passed the coffee shop, which was crowded with people talking happily. Smells of toasting bagels, coffee, and frying eggs drifted out. Still, Barbara said it was an emergency, so I passed it by.

Barbara was walking out of her office. She glanced down the hall, took my arm, and pulled me inside. She held a paper bag. I reached for it.

"Thanks for the coffee."

"It's not coffee," she whispered into my ear. She pulled a clear plastic urine specimen bottle from the bag. It contained muddy, dark-green liquid.

"Jesus, Barb, I can't imagine what this patient has. Looks like really deep jaundice."

"It's not urine. This is what the hospital water looked like most of the night. When the morning shift arrived, they called me. I found every nursing station had green water. It was in the drinking fountains, the sinks, and the toilets."

"What about the hemodialysis unit?" I asked. Booth had the biggest hemodialysis unit in New York City. It took little imagination to picture what would happen if the green water got into the dialysis machines. I felt a sheen of sweat on my forehead. We'd need to move fast, but I didn't know our next move.

Barbara said, "I called them. They said the water from the hospital system was green, but it turned clear after they filtered it."

"Why didn't the nurses call you last night?"

"The night administrator forbade the night staff from telling anybody. He said they would take care of it. Whatever they did, the water looks pretty clear this morning, but I'm anxious that some of the green stuff is still in the water. I tried some, and it tasted a little off, so I spit it out."

"People were drinking this last night?"

"Of course not. The nurses are only allowing people to drink bottled water."

"This is bad. I can't face it without that cup of coffee you promised. Let's talk about it in the coffee shop."

She drew her head back and swept her arms around me. I thought it was a hug, but she gripped me tightly, more like a python than my mother. Through her teeth, she said, "The whole hospital is falling apart, and you're worried about coffee?"

"Considering what we're faced with, I need two cups of coffee. Big ones. A bagel with cream cheese would be good, too."

"Who knows what kind of water they're using? We can't afford to lose you until this crisis is over."

"Thanks for the vote of confidence."

She ignored me. "Peggy's making a sweep through the hospital and collecting water samples from every floor."

"So nobody's drinking the water, right?"

"Well, I told the nurses. I don't have the authority over anyone else."

"Who does?"

"Carolyn. Let's go."

As we walked through the lobby, a woman held a little kid up to the drinking fountain. "Stop!" Barbara shrieked and lunged for the child. The mother pulled the kid close and hurried out the front door.

Shit, many people might be drinking contaminated water —a lot of them. Something in my chest clenched like a fist. I could feel us tipping into disaster.

Barbara led me in a fast walk into the executive suite. A fan of grand entrances, she tapped on Carolyn's door, then threw it open. We hurried in. Barbara pulled the door closed behind us. Barbara had known Carolyn Fulton, the hospital's deputy director, for years. She was the only administrator Barbara and I trusted.

Carolyn stood. "Close the door behind you, please." Carolyn was a tall, broad-shouldered woman with clear gray eyes that matched her cropped gray hair.

She said, "Thank you, Barbara, for alerting me to this problem. I instructed the administrator in charge of the physical plant to do whatever you tell him. He put up a fight at first, but he's neutralized now, the idiot. He'll do what you tell him.

"The physical plant supervisor is in his office. He thinks he knows what happened. He's waiting for you right now."

I took a breath. "Ms. Fulton, until we know what made the water green and if it's still contaminated, I think we'd better not let people drink it."

"Already done. We won't let anybody drink it until you give us medical clearance."

As tension left my muscles, I almost smiled. I said, "Thank you, Ms. Fulton. You and Barbara are stars."

"No need for thanks. Just tell me what's right, and I'll make it happen."

The maintenance office was in a corner of the basement. The director, Bob Schwartz, sat at his desk near the center of a big open office littered with cleaning machines, stacks of wood and drywall, and other junk. His desk was covered with forms, checklists, and work orders, many stained with oil or grease. When he rose to meet us, we saw he wore blue jeans and a brown shirt. A pretied necktie hung looped over his desk lamp. It seemed to have a greenish tinge. He looked to be in pain. His staff noisily walked in and out, clocking in and taking their machines. They were drinking coffee from a pot on a table.

"Am I glad to see you," he said and shook our hands. "I feel terrible about this."

"What exactly happened?"

"Around midnight, the night administrator woke me up because the nurses were complaining and asking questions. I came in and checked the connections and found both the potable water and antifreeze valves were open. It looked like antifreeze was getting into the potable water, the stuff you drink. The water turned green because the antifreeze discolored it. We turned the taps off and flushed the system. When the water was clear, I called my administrator, and he ordered the taps opened so people could drink.

"He said there are at least a thousand people in the building now, and we can't function without water. He told me if we had kept the water off, we would have to evacuate the patients and close down. People might die, and the hospital would lose millions, maybe even our accreditation."

"How, exactly, did the antifreeze get into the water?" I asked.

"Well, we've had this guy, Old Charley, for twenty or

thirty years. He isn't too bright and can't read many words, but he can do numbers real nice. He hardly has anything to do, but we keep him on because he loves it and brightens things up. You should see him smile when he makes the coffee in the morning. He always brings me the first cup."

"Did Charley make this coffee?" Barbara asked.

"No, I did. I rinsed everything out with the clear water."

I realized I'd be seeing green in liquids for years.

"After I was up all night with my staff, my administrator came in this morning and told me he's 'very disappointed with us.' Pretty clear he's throwin' me under the bus. Somebody's got to take the blame."

Barbara straightened, hands on her hips. "So you're throwing the rest of us under the bus?"

"Of course not. Easy, let's settle down. I'll tell you the whole thing."

"Did Charley drink antifreeze?" Barbara asked.

"No. Here's the deal. In the summer, the air conditioning system cools the water and pumps it around the building. In the fall, we add antifreeze to keep it from icing up."

I asked, "Why not keep antifreeze in it all year."

"Corrodes the pipes and shortens their life.

"When I called the foreman from the afternoon shift, he said nothing unusual happened except they put antifreeze into the air conditioning water. It's easy. You open one valve to drain the dirty water out of the system, then you turn the valve next to it to put in fresh. Then you close that valve and open the one next to it to let in the antifreeze. Finally, you close the antifreeze valve, and you're ready for winter."

"Were they labeled?" I said.

"Of course, but Charley doesn't read too well. He knew which was which, but when he finished, he forgot and left both the potable water and the air conditioner water open. That's how antifreeze got into the drinking water."

Barbara stared. "There's a valve that connects the air conditioning fluid to the potable water?"

"No. In any place the city water connects to the air conditioning system or a sewer, the law says the drinking water must be at higher pressure to prevent contamination from leaking into the potable system. There must be a backflow preventer to be sure the clean water supply pressure never falls below the contaminated water. That ensures we always have one-way flow from the drinking water into the other systems, never the other way."

"So what happened?" I asked.

"Nothing at first. About a half hour after they changed the valves, the nursing supervisor called and said they weren't letting anybody drink the water. That's when I told him to keep flushing out the system until we could straighten things out."

Barbara gradually moved right up to him and was maybe six inches from his face. She was either planning to sock him or strangle him.

I put a hand on each of their shoulders and pulled them apart.

"Let's see this plumbing," Barbara ordered.

We were in a world of hurt.

We took a freight elevator up to the mechanical floor just below the roof.

It was dark. Motors cycled on and off. We followed Bob in, and a curtain of feathery spiderwebs brushed into my hair and stuck. He turned on a switch. A few old incandescent bulbs winked on from the ceiling. It was hard to see in the dim light. Bob pulled a flashlight from a shelf near the door. Pipes covered the walls, and electrical wires of all sizes snaked in all directions.

"The building was built in 1957, and we've expanded dozens of times over the years. Each time we get in a different plumbing contractor. Lowest bidder. Each takes the blueprints for the system and marks where they've changed it. They sometimes don't understand what the last guys did, or they need to do something like raise the pressure when we added the top floors. If they find what they think is a mistake, they correct it."

He pulled a pack of cigarettes out of his pants pocket, pulled one out, and started to light it.

Then he noticed Barbara staring at him. "This is a nonsmoking building."

"Not up here." He pointed to an old oil can full of butts.

"It is now."

He put his cigarette back in the pack.

We stepped over empty cans and boxes of screws and bolts as Bob led us to the scene of the crime—a bank of levers and round valves like you see on outdoor spigots. A yellowing card hung over each, identifying its purpose.

I slid my hands down the dirty pipes. They were covered with black and gray dust and real spiderwebs, but nothing was there. "Where's the backflow preventer?"

He shined his light, fell to one knee, and finally lay on his back and scooted under the pipes. His hair must have felt filthy and creepy.

"Well, I'll be damned. There isn't one. God knows how long this has been open, just waiting for somebody to open both pipes at the same time." He paused. "Of course, there's no reason to do that, ever."

I asked, "Is this where the dialysis unit gets water from?"

"Inpatient dialysis is on the hospital system. Outpatient dialysis has its own water system because they're in a separate building."

Thank God.

"I have an idea," Barbara said. "Call a plumber to come in right now and fix the cross-connection."

"Yes," I said, "and keep flushing the water system until we tell you to stop."

"Do you know what that means?"

"Oh, you bet we do."

He looked shaken. "How will you tell if there's any antifreeze in the water?"

I tried to smile. "We'll figure it out somehow."

CHAPTER 6
FINDING THE
FREEZING POINT

When we got back to Barbara's office, we found Peggy had deposited sample bottles labeled with times and ward numbers all over the desk and chair. Barbara loaded them into a cardboard box, and we headed to the chemistry lab.

The lab was huge, nearly the size of a basketball court. There must have been forty people working at benches surrounded by gleaming machines. Each machine had dozens of thin tubes sucking tiny droplets of blood or serum in for different tests. Red and green lights flickered on and off. It must have been hard to concentrate, as the air was filled with beeps that notified their human servants to deliver more blood or supplies.

Barb, who knew everybody, led me to the lab supervisor's desk and dropped the box on his desk.

"Mark, meet Chad." He was in his late twenties or early thirties, wearing jeans and a T-shirt under his white coat. Barbara smiled at the outline of his pecs under the image of a Salvation Army Santa Claus. He looked like we'd put a box of dead rats on his desk.

"I've seen a few of these," he said. "The water in our taps turned green, too. It won't screw up our tests because we use distilled water." He nodded his head to rows of enormous glass jugs along one wall. "Since the water turned green, we use distilled water for everything."

"What about making coffee?"

"We are today. There's a pot of fresh coffee right there. You're welcome to some."

I glared at Barbara. "I've been dying for a cup. I guess you forgot to send out for mine. And the bagel."

"Sorry," she mumbled. "I've been preoccupied with squiring you around and saving lives." Her dark brown eyes focused on me sharply.

"Well, there's that," I said. I walked over and poured two cups.

"Thanks," she said. "That's nice of you."

"They're both for me."

She smiled. I gave her one of my cups. We were a team. Together we sniffed our coffees. It seemed rude, but we couldn't help it.

Fortified, I pointed to our boxes of water. "It's contaminated with antifreeze. Can you test for it? I think the main ingredient is ethylene glycol."

"You need special reagents for that. We'll have to order them and set up the test. We're doing the next best thing. Freezing point determinations. If there's antifreeze, it won't freeze."

Made sense.

He led us to a cluster of techs. On the counter in front of them were two big glass beakers partially filled with crushed ice. Tucked inside each was a smaller empty beaker surrounded by crushed ice. Chad poured a bottle of distilled water into one small beaker and a sample of green water into the other. Then he dropped rod-shaped magnets about the size of a peanut into each.

"Magnetic stirrers," he said, and switched on machines under each beaker. They began to spin. "That way, we'll make sure the temperatures are even throughout the water." A minute later, he turned off the stirrers and put a thermometer in each beaker. When the temperatures finally stopped falling, he held them up.

The distilled water had formed an icy sludge. "The plain water freezes at exactly zero degrees centigrade—as you'd expect." He switched the thermometer to the green water. It was fifteen degrees below zero.

"Looks like there's still antifreeze," he said.

We called Carolyn and told her the bad news. Next, Barbara and I went to the ER to talk to Mark Henry, the hospital toxicologist. It's always awkward when I meet somebody whose first name is the same as mine. Mark Henry was a tall and undeniably handsome blond man with an immaculate shirt and tie visible under his starched, tailored white coat. I looked down at mine. There were purple stains on the sleeves from staining bacteria. Near the lapels, a gravy-colored stain revealed my eating habits. I felt a bit shabby.

Two big windows brightened the office. A couple of toxicology books and a pad of yellow legal paper covered with jottings lay on his big desk. He had a cup of green water on his desk. Floor-to-ceiling bookshelves held neat lines of books and thick binders. Piles of carefully stacked papers stood in a corner. His airy, bright office was about four times bigger than mine.

He stood up and stretched his long legs. "I talked to the physical plant people. They gave me the brand name of the antifreeze they use, and I called the company that makes it. It's a typical antifreeze formulation. The active ingredient is ethylene glycol. Unless you have a concentrated solution, the stuff is colorless and tasteless. They include the green dye to warn people."

I asked, "So what are the symptoms?"

"At first, it looks like you've been drinking too much alcohol. You get woozy and dizzy. Unless you are treated quickly, you'll end up in a coma with multisystem failure. Anybody up on the wards look like they're drunk?"

"No more than usual," Barbara said. Her sense of humor seemed to be returning.

There was a loud knock on the door, and the hospital lawyer, Marcia Boznango, peered in. Her sharp nose and bulging eyes swept the office. She had the sallow, pasty complexion of one who rarely leaves the dimness of her office. If someone had told me she was a vampire, I'd have considered it. She wore a polyester pantsuit with a pattern that reminded me of a carpet. I felt like I was in a cage with an enormous snake sniffing me.

Her voice was brittle and precise. "It is standard operating procedure that I am informed about anything that puts us at risk of a lawsuit. I assume you were about to call me."

"Not exactly," Mark Henry said, "but you were next on our list."

She handed us a page from a pile of Xeroxes. "Here are the legal parameters all staff will work within, including you.

"Number one, you will not discuss this with patients, visitors, or media without my express permission. In advance. In writing.

"Two, before you make any intervention or take any other action to deal with the water, I want to clear it before you begin.

"Three, you are under no circumstances to call the city's public health department about this."

Mark Henry rose, walked to the door, and shook her hand. "Rest assured that we'll keep you in the loop, Marcia. Now, if you'll excuse us, we'll wrap up this meeting." She spun and silently disappeared. She left the door to the noisy ER yawning open.

Mark and I looked at each other. I said, "Thank God

Marcia came in. The city will shut us down if they find out about this before we report it."

"Damn straight," Mark agreed.

We spent the next half hour on a conference call with city epidemiologists, laboratory experts, and water engineers. It turned out the city could run tests for ethylene glycol and give us accurate measurements.

The Chief City Water engineer said, "Provide us samples, and we'll test every hour. Until then, nobody drinks or uses the water. You must keep flushing water through the system until we tell you it's safe to drink."

"Absolutely," Mark said.

"Good," the city engineer said. "We'll have another conference call later in the day to discuss our progress."

Among the many great things about living in New York is that you can get special laboratory tests done instantly. The city personnel are knowledgeable and helpful. Barbara and I left the office, quietly closing the door. She headed back to the lab and administration to report on our plan and arrange to link up with the city lab.

I went to my office and sat down. I realized this was the first time I was relaxed all day. We'd defined the problem and made a plan. Now, all we had to do was follow the program. I felt great.

There was a sharp knock on my door.

"It's me, Peggy." She handed me a tuna sandwich with melted cheese and two cups of coffee. "I thought tuna would make a better lunch. I made sure they made the coffee with bottled water."

"What about the bagel?"

"I had to walk two blocks to a deli. They were out of bagels, so this is what you get."

"You're a star, Peggy. We make a great team."

She winked, smiled, and left.

I finally had time to make rounds on my patients. I paged my residents and told them to meet me in the ICU.

The senior resident on my service was a young doctor named Dominic Fererro.

He looked terrible. He stood slightly bent forward, sensitive brown eyes on the floor. The whites of his eyes were dull red.

"What's the matter?"

"Last night, I was called to see an old lady on hemodialysis. She had an anion gap, a big one. There had to be an unknown acid in her blood."

I said, "Only a few things cause that. It should be easy to figure out. Which one is it?"

Dominic said, "I ruled out all the causes except ethylene glycol poisoning."

"Oh, oh. I think I know where it came from."

"You're the only one who agrees with me. My lady was on dialysis. The treatment for ethylene glycol poisoning is dialysis, so she should have been getting better. Instead, she got worse. I called in the senior resident. He didn't believe me, even though he couldn't think of a likely cause. We asked other residents. None of them could figure it out either. Nobody believed me.

"After everybody left, I stayed at my lady's bedside. Her blood pressure fluctuated over the next hour, but the trend was down and down. Her pulse got thready, and it looked like she was getting a myocardial infarction. Her lungs failed, and I had to call anesthesia. They had a terrible time getting the tube into her trachea. She bucked and tried to wave her arms even though they were in restraints. She ended up on 100 percent oxygen. I woke up the renal fellow, but he wouldn't let me take her off the machine. It was a blessing when she lost consciousness."

"Dom, that green stuff in the water was antifreeze. Was the dialysis fluid green?"

"I don't think so."

"Time to get to dialysis."

We marched briskly to the dialysis unit. It could be a disaster if the day shift admitted more patients. When we arrived in the big room, all the machines were lined up against the walls. Our words seemed to disappear into the echoing silence. The head nurse picked up a phone and called the head of the dialysis program, Dr. Sheridan.

As always, his sonorous, deep Israeli voice was deadly serious. "Until we figure this out, I'm diverting all the patients to the outpatient dialysis unit. We can't take chances with all those lives. I've closed the inpatient unit until we can be certain there's no risk. It's a sacred trust to do no harm to our patients. And you know some of them are our friends."

"It's ethylene glycol," I said. "Mark Henry says ethylene glycol is a tiny molecule that goes through filters. They put in uridine green to mark the fluid so people will know not to drink it."

Dr. Sheridan cleared his throat. "For inpatient dialysis, we run the water through a series of filters that are so fine even viruses can't get through them, though tiny molecules like ethylene glycol can. The uridine green is a large molecule. Since the water after the filters was clear, I assume the uridine green was caught there.

"For years, we've been asking the hospital for a reverse osmosis system. That will take everything out of the water so we're sure it's pure. But you know how tight these Salvationists on the board of directors can be."

I didn't know, of course. I didn't travel in the powerful circle that Sheridan did.

He said, "Thank God, there was only one patient last night. It could have been like a terrorist attack—dead people everywhere. I've got another call."

Like the royalty he was, he dismissed me.

The dialysis nurse took us to the offending machine. From

the way she looked at it, I was surprised it wasn't surrounded by crime scene tape. Then she took us to the water filter.

"Where's the chart?" Dominic asked. Dry-eyed and competent, he was back in his groove. Thank God.

"The chart? Barbara, I mean Mrs. Russo, took it."

"Thanks, we'll read it with her."

We walked down the hall to the elevator. The doors opened, and Marcia swept out, eyes ahead. She didn't seem to see us as she steamed down the hall to the dialysis center.

Dominic said, "I'd love to see her face when she finds out we got the chart before she could hide it."

Barbara's office was empty. We found her copying the last pages of the chart at a copier in the back of the 3-West nursing floor, where Marica would never look for her.

As she raised her head, her smile radiated pleasure. "I heard Marcia was after the chart. So I decided to make us a copy before it gets lost."

"Barb, you are six of the seven wonders of the modern world."

The patient turned out to be ninety-two years old and schizophrenic. She wanted to die and had to be forced to take medicines and hemodialysis to keep her alive against her will. The dialysis nurses' notes said this was the first time she hadn't fought to get off the machine. One of the notes said, "her psychotherapy finally seems to be working."

In retrospect, it was an overly optimistic interpretation.

For the rest of the day, we sent a messenger with a water sample to the city lab every hour to the city lab to test for ethylene glycol. By 6:00 p.m., the ethylene glycol was at undetectable levels. The lab guy said the water was now below the legal limit.

We flushed the water system for two more hours and then opened it up for general use.

What a day. I made my way back to Manhattan and pulled up to our little apartment on West 113th Street. I told Jessica about it. She shook her head, walked into the kitchen, and got me a beer.

I was on my second when the phone rang. The caller had such a loud voice I had to hold the phone away from my ear.

"I'm in charge of epidemiology for Queens."

"Nice to meet you. What can I do for you?"

"I've already called your hospital. I'm closing it down. You will need to transfer all the patients to other hospitals. We must put patient safety first, and until I am satisfied, the hospital is closed. Now."

I felt like Bill Murray in the movie *Ghostbusters* when he meets Mr. Peck, the jerk from the EPA.

"But your own lab says the water is safe. I have the levels right here."

"It's my decision, not yours. I've got a lot of other calls to make, so I have to hang up."

"If you do, my first call will be to the *New York Times*, then the other papers and TV stations."

"You wouldn't dare."

"Why not? Imagine the headlines. If we're lucky, we'll both be on the news shows. We'll be famous."

"You'll be hearing from me again. Soon." The bang from his hanging up hurt my ear even though I held the phone away from my head.

I called Barbara. She got hold of the administration and canceled the closing.

In the end, the hemodialysis unit got its reverse osmosis system. I meant to check with the physical plant people to see what happened to Old Charley. They probably retired him.

I hope they ordered out for coffee at his party.

CHAPTER 7
FELILIA MANEJA MENDOZA

Things settled down after the antifreeze incident. I always started morning rounds by checking on bacterial cultures in the microbiology lab, then led my residents up the stairs to the Respiratory ICU on the eighth floor. The rest of the day, we'd percolate down from floor to floor, seeing our patients. On each floor, I got a new Styrofoam cup of vile coffee, which meant at least eight cups a day, five or six days a week, for six years.

I loved to make the residents climb up the stairs with me. It proved I still had it in me. I loved the soft morning light pouring in through the windows of the Respiratory ICU. Most of all, I loved seeing Miss Mendoza, who usually joined us as we walked from patient to patient. Typically, the nurse assigned to that patient provided their report, then the intern and resident, and then I'd examine the patient, review the chart, and critique and teach.

Miss Mendoza inserted herself right before me and made her own summary. She was smart and focused. She called 'em like she saw 'em and was unafraid to take on any doctor, including the heads of the surgery and medicine departments. She liked stirring up trouble.

Everybody watched themselves around her except for a privileged few. I knew I was in this golden circle my first week when she told me her nickname. Everyone in the Philippines has a nickname, some of which sound funny to Americans, like Ballsy or Bong Bong. Miss Mendoza's nickname was Budsy.

If Budsy liked you, she would take care of your patients' respirators, draw blood gases, and make adjustments to correct any problems. Nurses weren't technically allowed to interpret blood gases, so she was supposed to call. If she didn't like you, she might ring you every half hour, even at night—especially at night.

Doctors could sleep in a little on-call room across the hall from the unit. A big bell hung on the wall. If you pissed off the nurses, they would lean on the bell at 4:00 a.m.

On rounds, my entire team would sometimes wait for her to go ahead of us to watch her walk. Oh, that little white dress. She turned and smiled back with those lovely dark eyes, and I was sure—well, pretty sure—she was smiling at me.

I thought a lot about those smiles. It had been six years since my first wife, Bobbie, left me. I went out occasionally, but loving Bobbie was in my soul. I couldn't fully love anybody else. I lived for a couple of years with Jessica, a wonderful woman. Every time I'd feel a flush of love for her, Bobbie would pop into my mind. In the end, I left Jessica. A sad and miserable day for both of us.

Then one morning, I was standing in the sunny kitchen of my apartment, eating a piece of toast with peanut butter for breakfast. I realized something was gone. Staring out the window into the lovely warm golden morning light, I realized I no longer loved Bobbie.

Sad to admit, this was one of the high points of my life. This was the second time I had made a great life discovery while eating peanut butter on toast. When things get tough, I head for the PB.

That morning, I asked Budsy if I could take her to dinner. She accepted and gave me her address.

She lived on the top floor of an old white house a few blocks from the hospital. I was nervous as I walked up the stairs. A pile of phone books was stacked inside the door. I picked them up and wobbled up the steps. Since my hands were full of books, I had to knock on the door with my forehead. In the middle of the third knock, she pulled the door open. I tumbled forward, dropping books at her feet. She wore a little blue tube dress. It seemed to be tenuously attached. She also wore a big smile and happy, deep-brown eyes. I leaned in and kissed her, a long, dreamy kiss. She stepped back against the wall. She felt warm and soft. Finally, she pulled her face back and took a breath. "I guess I should invite you in. I'll show you where to put the books."

I'd forgotten about them. She said, "That's a great way to start a date," and led me into the apartment.

The living room was filled with trees and flowing tropical vines. In the center was a thirty- or forty-gallon aquarium filled with large, undistinguished-looking gray fish.

"You can put the phone books next to the tank. These are my piranhas. Because you're my special guest, I'll let you feed them." She dipped a net into a small goldfish aquarium and scooped one up.

"I name these after doctors." She smiled. "This one is that asshole cardiologist, Dr. Bowles." She handed me the net, and I dropped the little cardiologist in with the piranhas. Nothing happened. It swam nervously among the big fish.

"Have you ever named one after me?"

"Not yet."

"Is there something wrong with the goldfish?"

"No, the piranhas usually wait until I'm gone. Then they strike."

I kissed her again.

It was a good date. A great date. Outstanding. I remember asking if she'd teach me Tagalog, the language of the Philippines.

"Sure," she said.

"How do I say, 'I love you?'"

"Funny you should ask. If you love someone like a sister or brother, it's *mahal ko*. It's like, 'You're dear to me.'"

I asked the obvious question. "How about 'I want to make love to you?'"

"Well, *Iniibig kita* means I love you romantically."

"Is that like, 'I want to screw you?'"

"You've got no class. There's no way of saying that in my language. We use the English word. You know, we describe our history as four hundred years in a convent with the Spanish and a hundred years in a whorehouse with the Americans."

"I'll try to do better."

"Good. Let me show you the bedroom."

We had a long, amazing night.

When we eventually returned to the living room, the goldfish was gone, but a little cloud of golden yellow scales drifted in the water. "Looks like we're too late," she said.

The next morning, she made breakfast of fish and rice with eggs. I ate fish and rice at least once a day for the next thirteen years. After six years, I got to like it.

The following day, she wasn't at work. Of course, I didn't ask, but I wondered if this had anything to do with our date. By noon, I was beside myself. I called a florist and sent her a dozen roses. She wasn't in the ICU the next day either, so I sent another dozen. I asked my partner, Barbara Berger, a practical Brooklynite, for advice. She was very different from Barbara Russo, in a good way. You can never know too many Barbaras.

"I'm sure she's delighted. Quit wasting money. I know

where we can get roses wholesale." She drove me to get them and watched me run up Budsy's sidewalk, lay the roses on the threshold, and ring her doorbell. Then I rushed back out to Barbara's car.

"Time to go, Barb."

"She'll be out in a second."

"Exactly, let's go." Barbara drove so slowly. The car was still in second gear as we passed the end of Budsy's block. I focused my attention on the hood of the car and tried to calm my breathing without being too obvious.

The next night, Budsy called me. Presumably, Barbara gave her the number.

"Quit sending me roses. Don't waste money." Something in her tone might mean she felt we might be sharing finances soon. My heart bounded. "Would you like to have dinner tonight?" she asked.

"With you?"

"Don't be dense. See you in two hours."

She was beyond beautiful when she opened the door. I could smell dinner cooking. She served crabs, fish, and rice.

She politely asked me if I needed help opening the crabs.

I thought of eating crabs in Baltimore—big tables covered with newspapers and wooden hammers to break the shells. "I love to crack crabs. Bring 'em on."

She didn't have any hammers, so I ate rice as we talked. Finally, she got up and showed me how to open a crab shell with a fork. It was delicious.

After a delightful evening, I felt it was time to get serious. We were holding each other. I looked into her deep-brown eyes. "Budsy, what's your mother's name?"

"Illuminada. Why do you ask?"

"What name did she give you?"

She smiled. "Nobody asks me that. I'm Felilia Maneja Mendoza."

"Felilia Maneja Mendoza, will you marry me?"

"It took you long enough. Yes."

"I wanted to be sure."

She smiled sleepily. "Then let's go to bed."

We slept together for the rest of her life.

CHAPTER 8
WEDDING BELLS AND
SUCKLING PIGS

A couple of days after I moved in with Budsy, she looked up from her plate of fish stuffed with raisins and asked, "When are you going to announce our engagement?"

I swallowed. "Doesn't the girl do that?"

"Not this girl." Her look and voice were intent.

"I'll make the announcement tomorrow." I had no idea what to do. I pictured dozens of embarrassing conversations. "You're marrying Budsy?" or "You're kidding, right?" or "Do you know who she was dating before you?" or "My sister would be perfect for you. She's a doctor, and she likes you," etc. Before the day was out, I heard them all. Except it was two brothers who wanted me to marry their sister.

In the end, I put the announcement on the opening screen of all the computers in the Department of Medicine. I'd been programming the system as a favor to Internal Medicine, and it gave me some perks.

Some friends wished us well. Others smiled or giggled. I was climbing a back staircase when I ran into an Indian guy who'd dated Budsy on and off for years. He looked sourly down at me and said, "You move fast, don't you?"

I looked up and said, "Sunil, I know what I want." And I did.

Barbara Berger had known what was coming ever since she helped me buy roses. She was a real friend. Barbara trained at Downstate, which specialized in sexually transmitted diseases. She wrote a classic paper on STDs in gay women. They rarely get anything aside from chlamydia, which she called "clams." What an image. She offered to advise me on where to get good cheap wedding rings, but I already had a plan.

I told Budsy, "Here's the deal. I bought Bobbie's engagement ring for sixty-eight dollars. Let's go down to the jewelry district, and I'll spend ten times as much on you."

Her eyes softened. "How sweet." The next day I drove her to Manhattan, and we traipsed from store to store. Each salesperson conveyed the same wordless message: "I don't offer discounts, but maybe for you . . ."

Finally, Budsy smiled and said, "Before we make a decision, let's check with my jewelry guy."

Holy shit, she had a jewelry guy.

She directed me to Brooklyn, where we stopped at a dirty beige high-rise that looked so old it might collapse. The jeweler's apartment was on the thirty-fifth floor. The jeweler had blond hair, pale eyes, and no smile.

Budsy said, "Ivan, this is my fiancé, Mark. We want to look at a wedding ring."

"What do you have in mind?"

She took a pad from her purse and sketched a tall diamond on a golden ring. "One or two carats will do just fine."

Blood drained from my brain as I saw how much money would soon be drained from my bank account. She and the Russian negotiated for a few minutes. Then she asked me to write him a check for $2,000. Overwhelmed that it was not more, I scribbled the check. He threw in a wedding ring for me, too.

In the elevator, she said, "It was cheap because I accept flaws that can't be seen with the naked eye."

Smart girl. I asked how she came to have a jewelry guy.

"He was a patient and noticed I like to wear lots of jewelry." Gold looked lovely with her brown skin. "He asked if he could make me some stuff for me to sell. If a nurse or visitor compliments me on a piece of jewelry, I take it off and sell it for cash right there. I've made a lot of money." She opened her purse and held up a set of those fitting rings jewelers use to find your size. "I do the same thing with clothes."

I was pleased to marry a thrifty immigrant.

Over the following months, we began to learn how to live together. It started with smoking. Occasionally, she'd pull out a cigarette and puff away.

"Buds, I can't see myself married to a woman who smokes."

"I'll stop, but you'll have to stop something, too."

"Like what?"

"Coffee. By the end of the morning, you have a tremor."

I'd never noticed the tremor, but there it was. No wonder my handwriting was so lousy. I quit for years.

Budsy's one indulgence was that she drove a chocolate-colored Toyota Supra, a rakish, low-slung fastback sports car. It was incredibly expensive. A couple of weeks after we bought the ring, she parked it in Brooklyn, and somebody stole it in broad daylight.

That night, she dug the papers out of a drawer. It turned out she was leasing it. The agreement had a big box in bold font saying that if anything happened to the car, including theft, she agreed to pay the remaining payments. She had initialed the box. This could cost tens of thousands of dollars, and she still wouldn't have a car. It seemed we were hosed, but it also seemed so iniquitous that I spent a couple of hours fighting with the leasing agency. I eventually talked them down to $800.

The next day, I drove her to a Chrysler dealer. In the center of the showroom sat a Mitsubishi Conquest, a sexy little red fastback. The price was reasonable, so I took it for a drive. As soon as we got back, I wanted to be sure she was comfortable in the driver's seat.

The salesman, a swarthy fellow, said, "Go ahead, honey, and take a test drive, too."

She smiled. "I can't drive a stick."

The salesman stared at her, then back at me. His lip curled. He laughed. He addressed the showroom. "This guy is buying a sports car for a woman who can barely reach the accelerator. She can't even drive a stick!"

We left.

I must have left my name and phone number because the sales manager called that night. "I apologize for my employee. Come back and ask for me, and I'll make it right."

"No thanks," I said.

"I'll make it worth your while. You'll like the price."

The next day, I returned. The manager was a pleasant middle-aged guy, balding, and quite a few pounds over-weight. I wouldn't have been surprised if he'd had a cigar jutting from the corner of his mouth.

He walked me to the car and pointed to the price sticker on the window.

He pointed his stubby finger at the Manufacturer's Suggested Retail Price, about $25,000. "The number over here is the wholesale cost of the car—what I paid for it." It was $3,000 less than the retail price.

"To make up for your bad experience, I'll sell it to you for a thousand dollars below wholesale."

My spidey sense told me something was wrong. "You're telling me you're taking a loss?" I felt sarcasm and suspicion in my voice. "How can you make money doing this?"

"I sell a lot of cars, and they give me rebates. I'm still making a profit. Don't worry about me; send your friends."

Budsy and I drove the streets near our house for the next week. She was a fast learner, but it was not a smooth process. Once, the car was jerking uncontrollably toward a parked car. "Brakes!" I shrieked.

She stopped. I smelled the clutch burning. Uncharacteristically, she said, "I'm sorry." This happened many times. Rinse and repeat as needed. Notably, she once stalled out in the middle of an intersection. "You take over," she said through tears and gritted teeth.

I pulled her back into the seat. "No way. You can do this."

She jerked out of the intersection, pulled over, got herself together, and drove home without problems. A tough cookie she was, and I loved it. A week later, she was tooling around town like a pro, leaving rubber whenever she saw a friend.

We hadn't heard the last of her old car. The guys who stole the Supra drove it around the city and parked it illegally, ignoring the fines. Periodically, the city sent us irate letters. I had to go to the police station to show the documentation that we'd reported it stolen so they would cancel the fines. Otherwise, they'd take the money out of my bank account. You'd think that if they got close enough to put a ticket on the car, they'd have checked to see if it was stolen.

Taking Budsy to Michigan to meet my family led to an interesting exchange. My brother picked us up at the airport and drove to my parents' home, where everybody awaited us in the living room.

My dad said, "Budsy, I'd like to welcome you to our family."

She bowed her head slightly. "I'm so glad to finally meet you."

A few minutes of chitchat followed, then she looked at me. "Get me a glass of water."

This would not stand. I showed her who was boss. "No."

Aghast, the family sat in silence.

She smiled nicely and held my eyes. "Get me a glass of water, or I'll cut off your balls."

Everyone laughed. My dad almost fell out of his chair. He reached over and squeezed her arm.

"Two cubes," she said.

I got her the water. And the two ice cubes.

Then it was back to Flushing. While she was running the ICU, I saw some interesting cases. Periodically, the Salvationists felt the need to serve some of the truly needy and sent a truck to the Bowery to pick up a few poor characters to import to the hospital. One day, they brought in a guy who worked delousing people. The ER docs called me.

The guy sat on a cart, shaking with chills. His temperature was 104 degrees, and he had a severe headache. He looked like he had chickenpox, with bumps clustering mostly on his body and upper arms.

"What happened?" I asked.

"I got some nasty-assed bug bite on my leg. It turned black. About a week later, I got the pox."

He held up his light leg, and I saw a black hole in his ankle about the size of a dime. Thin pus flowed down toward his foot. "That's an eschar," I told him.

"What's that?"

I said, "A dry hole in your skin. Only a few diseases cause eschars, so it'll help figure out what's wrong."

Measles was out because its rash is flat. Rocky Mountain Spotted Fever was possible, but it doesn't have a black scab. The most important disease to rule out was syphilis. You can get an ulcer with syphilis, but it's usually on the genitals, and it isn't black. Also, the rash likes the hands and feet, where it's cooler.

That left Kew Gardens fever as the most likely diagnosis.

Kew Gardens is a neighborhood a few miles from our hospital. The disease is caused by rickettsia, odd organisms that are halfway between viruses and bacteria. The most famous one is *Rickettsia rickettsia*, which causes Rocky Mountain spotted fever. *Rickettsia akari* causes Kew Gardens fever. You get the disease after being bitten by a tiny mite, a kind of chigger.

"Sir, I think you were bitten by a tiny mite that likes to live on mice."

"You can treat me, right?"

"Yes. I'll give you some tetracycline, and you should be fine."

My favorite rickettsia is *Rickettsia tsutsugamushi*, which causes scrub typhus.

My patient called a few days later to tell me he was fine. Nice to know.

Budsy scheduled our wedding for the end of summer with the reception following in a hotel out on Long Island. It turned out to be the day of the World Series. Still, my closest friends, Smelly Mellie Hochman, head of the Medical ICU, and surgeons Jim Turner and Kenny Rifkind, showed up. Real menches.

I had always found the waterfall of thick black hair running down Budsy's back thrilling. I later learned this meant she was available. The day before the wedding, she cut it into a pixie style that made her look like an impossibly charming Asian fairy. She set a circlet of orchids and jasmine around her head like a queen. What a beauty.

Bobbie had bought our little boys' suits for the occasion, and they zipped around the apartment like little blond mice. Every time the phone rang, Budsy answered. After the third call, she laughed. "It was your ex. I knew she'd call and try to screw things up."

"How'd you know?"

"I'm a woman. An experienced woman."

We were married by the hospital chaplain. It turns out that everyone in the Salvation Army can legally marry people, so we were wed in the hospital chapel. The bridal party entered the ER and proceeded up the stairs to the chapel while patients and staff gawked. My brother took dozens of pictures.

We drove out to Long Island for lunch. Mel and the surgeons had called ahead to ask the hotel to place a TV in the back of the room so they could keep one foot in the sports world and one in the reception.

CHAPTER 9
THE NATIONAL SPORT

We settled into married life. Budsy found a better job supervising all the ICUs at Maimonides Hospital in Brooklyn. I was nervous somebody might steal her new little sports car, but she only parked in the hospital lot, so it was always there at the end of the day.

A year later, Barbara Russo tapped on my office door. She was in her power sweater, dark crimson with large white letters spelling "BRA" across the front. She said it stood for her initials, Barbara Russo Antonelli, but I think it was because she was proud of her ample figure.

"I had a talk with Carolyn. May I sit down?"

I rushed to clear books and articles from my visitor chair. I said, "That's nice. How's life in the executive suite?"

She sat distractedly.

"Thanks. The women are still all Irish and wear polyester pantsuits. That's not why I'm here. Carolyn wants to know if Budsy would be willing to come back and set up a discharge planning department. I agree with Carolyn that she has the personality and the passion."

"What's discharge planning?"

She grimaced. "Many AIDS patients can't leave because

nobody wants to be near them. They often can't find apartments because landlords are afraid to rent to them.

"It costs us over three hundred dollars to keep a patient in a single-bed room. Once they are well enough to go home, insurance companies won't pay for the hospital room. We can't throw them out in the street, even though we lost over a million dollars in the last six months alone. Worse, there are fewer beds for paying patients who need surgery or short-term care, so we lose millions more. We'll have to close in six months unless we can free up beds."

I saw her point. "Sounds like a problem, all right. How could Budsy help?"

Barbara took a deep breath. "Budsy's job, if she takes it, will be to arrange for home care and nag landlords to rent apartments to AIDS patients. It's much cheaper for the hospital, even if we pay the rent ourselves."

"God knows Budsy's ambitious. She might miss clinical work. You know she's in charge of six ICUs at Maimonides."

Barbara stood. "Department heads make much more than nursing supervisors. Her job will pay more than most department heads."

I said, "She'll never wear a polyester pantsuit." Budsy was a delightfully flamboyant dresser with bright colors, tight dresses, and short skirts.

"I think Buds will do a great job. She's more likely to take the job if Carolyn offers it than you or me."

That night, Budsy burst through the door with a big smile and said, "I had a meeting with Carolyn. She says she might have a job for me. It's a promotion, and I'll make more money than the Head of the Nursing Department.

Budsy walked into her big new office a month later and began recruiting staff. She also began kicking ass and taking names. It didn't take long to wear down the home care agencies, landlords, and social services to the point that they were afraid to argue and just conceded whatever she wanted.

Unlike Budsy, I was in trouble. All the HIV patients were burning me out. Part of it was that most patients were my age or younger and middle class, like me. You expect old people to die, but young ones dying hit you hard.

A few months later, I cleaned up one of the piles of mail on my desk and found an official-looking letter from CDC. They were looking for a consultant to work for the Philippine government of Corazon Aquino. I could leave all the AIDS behind and move to the Philippines.

I had to get to Manila immediately. There was only one problem: The letter was dated two months ago, and the applications had closed two weeks ago.

I picked up the phone and called the number in Atlanta. A crabby voice answered. "Applications are closed."

"I know we are past the deadline, but I'd appreciate it if you'll consider me anyway."

"I'll keep you in mind," the voice said with heavy insincerity.

"I'll fax my CV."

"Suit yourself."

Two days later, Stan Music, head of the Division of International Health at CDC, called. "I delegated this hire to Jerry, and he convinced himself you weren't serious."

Stan was my boss for several years. He revealed his eccentricity when CDC sent him to study at the London School of Hygiene and Tropical Medicine. He returned wearing a brushy mustache and a bowler hat, carrying an umbrella.

Years later, when I became head of the Division of International Health, I found the files. As I expected, I was the only applicant for the Philippine job.

The US Agency for International Development (USAID) was funding the job. They booked Budsy and me in business class, and we cruised across the Pacific in the top compartment of a 747 as attendants stuffed us with champagne and caviar.

Budsy smiled and said, "I'm feeling better about this already."

We landed and fought our way through the steamy airport. Budsy's sister and brother-in-law waited outside. They loaded us into a homemade ice truck made of tin or steel. It looked like they'd made it with an erector set.

The front of the famous Manila Hotel was impressive. Budsy's brother-in-law stopped on the street and climbed out to get our luggage.

Budsy said, "It's ten yards up the hill to the door. We're not going to walk all that way with three suitcases."

He said, "I'm afraid they'll chase me away."

"I'll tell my husband to deal with them." She smiled at me.

We chugged up the hill and creaked to a stop at the entrance. The doormen treated us with respect. I gave them a big tip. Our deluxe suite high in the Manila Hotel was one flight below where General McArthur had ruled the country. Buds felt even better.

"This calls for more champagne and caviar," I declared and called room service. As an afterthought, I asked how much it cost. It was $160. I reconsidered.

Ten minutes later, a waiter tapped on the door with our beer and peanuts.

I tipped him two dollars, a lot of money at that time.

The time difference between the Philippines and the US is twelve hours, but we were too excited to sleep until sometime after 4:00 a.m.

At 8:00 a.m. on the dot, my counterpart and soon-to-be best friend and boss tapped on the door. "Hi, I'm Manolet Dayrit, Head Executive Assistant to Dr. Bengzon, the Secretary of Health." He was a handsome man, strong and fit, with a blazing white smile. Newspapers called it "the famous

Dayrit smile." Manolet had a great sense of humor. He was intelligent, passionate, and driven to improve people's health. He later became Secretary of Health for the Philippines, then Director of the Division of Human Capital for the World Health Organization (WHO). When he retired, he returned to Manila and took over as Dean of Ateneo Medical School, which Filipinos like to point out was founded by the Spanish five hundred years before Harvard.

He loaded me into an ancient little green Ford and gave me a tour of parts of the vast city of Manila. As we drove around, he prepared me for the job interview.

"Dr. Bengzon developed a negative attitude toward Americans because you supported Marcos in the years he was oppressing us." Filipinos always seemed to say "you" when they meant the American government, as though I was president for the previous twenty years. I was too tired and freaked out to correct him.

Manolet continued, "Many of his friends were tortured or killed, and he's skeptical that American doctors have anything to teach us. He thinks you're all spies."

"With all due respect, Manolet, who'd want to spy on a health department?"

"He's also in charge of kicking out the American bases or negotiating the price up to hundreds of millions of dollars. He's a man of principle, but we need the money badly. Marcos cratered the economy, and we need to build things up fast, so people don't go hungry."

I rubbed my eyes. Manolet looked across the seat to be sure I was awake. "You don't need to worry much about jet lag. Dr. Bengzon will interview you at eight tonight so that it will be like eight in the morning for you."

I turned my bleary eyes to his. "Except I'll be awake all day. I'll be pretty strung out."

Changing the subject, Manolet said, "I was in the opposition, too. We were in Mindanao, living in the mountains."

"You don't seem to hate Americans."

"I admire CDC. I took a course there once. Our project was to do a survey. It was right after the seat belt law. We hid in the bushes by the parking lot and recorded the percentage of CDC employees wearing belts. It was about 20 percent. I presented it to the head of the Bureau of Epidemiology, and they loved it.

"Dr. Bengzon thinks Marcos would have been overthrown decades ago without the billions in American aid. Nearly all the American support went straight to Marcos, his army, and his cronies. As best as I can tell, none trickled down to the rest of us.

"We have epidemics and outbreaks all over the place. We need to be able to prevent these to improve the health of the people." It sounded left-wing, but I liked how it focused on a clear goal. I've followed it ever since.

"We need to build the capacity to stop disease, and CDC is the only place in the world that has it. I convinced Dr. Bengzon to invite CDC in general and you in particular."

"I see." I could barely see because I was so tired. I tried to pretend I was awake.

Manolet pulled over and stopped the car. He twisted in his seat and looked me in the eye. "Last week, we interviewed the first American consultant. He seemed OK to most of us. Dr. Bengzon is a neurologist, and he gave the guy a psychological test. The guy gave all the wrong answers. Not only did he not offer the guy a job, but he referred him to a psychiatrist."

"Holy shit." I was awake now.

"I'll help you memorize the answers. "The first is 'yellow,' then 'three.' The next one is 'I want to be director of the play,' then 'ask a policeman,' then 'green,' 'ninety-nine,' 'the sister with the black hair,' 'move the truck three feet' and 'put the chair in the empty parking space.'"

Of course, I instantly forgot everything except "green" and "yellow."

"The Department of Health is across town, so I'll pick you up at six. Traffic is always terrible."

He dropped me back at the hotel, where I lay in bed and stared at the ceiling. This felt like a calamity in the making. I couldn't sleep. Budsy ordered me a steak and two beers. A typical last meal.

Manolet finally picked me up for the interview. The moon sent sickly shafts through the murky atmosphere. This time we drove into the vast, dim slums of Tondo, where narrow streets were lined with old wooden buildings collapsing from termites. Basketball nets blocked off many streets. I glanced at a group of men in red shirts carrying red flags running down a distant road.

Manolet said, "Don't worry, it's just the NPA, New People's Army. After we won the revolution, all the middle-class people came down from the mountains. There's only a rump left fighting the government, mostly criminals."

We soon came to the tall white walls of San Lazaro Hospital, one of the world's great fever hospitals. The Spanish built it in 1577, and people have been adding buildings ever since. Manolet drove us through a gate and into the complex.

We got out, and Manolet pointed at some big buildings. "That's the hospital. Over here is the Bureau of Labs, Chronic Diseases, and the National Capital Region Building. The secretary's office is in this two-story job in front of us."

The buildings were all painted white, inside and out. He led me to a waiting room. Soon, an assistant came out and led us in.

A long mahogany table filled most of the room. Dr. Bengzon—a large, broad-shouldered man—sat at the head. Along the sides sat undersecretaries and program managers. I stood alone at the foot. My head was a roiling mass of muddy thoughts. The colors, shapes, words, and numbers Manolet had forced me to memorize drifted around like sharp-edged icebergs on a frozen sea.

Dr. Bengzon welcomed me, then glanced down at my CV. "I see you were born in Detroit."

Here was one I could answer. "Yes, sir."

"What are the stats on the Detroit Pistons?"

"I don't know, sir. I'm not a sports guy."

Dr. Bengzon put down my CV and smiled. "The interview's over. You can hardly advise us if you don't know that basketball is our national sport."

Humiliated, I replied, "Thank you for considering me." I bowed my head and turned.

Manolet stood. "Wait! He plays *sung ka* (the national board game), and he's married to a Filipina."

"He might have said so," Dr. Bengzon said sourly. "Go see Mario."

Mario Taguiwalo was the undersecretary, the guy who made everything happen. He led Manolet and me to his office. Mario was what my mother called "portly." Unlike Dr. Bengzon, he had a great sense of humor.

"Welcome aboard. Did Manolet tell you about me?"

"Only your job." I was slowly shedding my panic and despair.

"I've had many jobs." Mario smiled, popping a delicious-smelling pork rind into his mouth. Seeing me staring, he pushed the package across his desk toward me.

"Most recently, I was head of propaganda for the New People's Army in the central islands, the Visayas. That's where I met Alran."

"Who's Alran?"

"Dr. Bengzon. His nickname is based on his initials, Alfredo RA Bengzon."

I crunched a pork rind.

"When things got hot under Marcos, I spent a few years managing a sports stadium in Saudi Arabia. I missed home, so I came back. My passion is acting, and I have played parts in dozens of movies. Unfortunately, directors limited me to playing heavies.

"In my favorite part, I played a jealous gangster. I followed my wife to her boyfriend's house and waited outside to confront them. As I sit steaming in the car, the camera makes a lovely tight close-up of my face. From behind me, a hand reaches around with a wicked knife and slits my throat. I squeeze a bulb, and fake blood pours in a sheet down my neck."

He smiled fondly. "Well, first thing in the morning, Manolet will take you to Personnel. The papers will be waiting for you there. Manolet will show you around. At noon, you'll interview applicants for the first class."

"Come on," Manolet said. "I'll show you our office." It turned out to be a big empty room. "I got it easily. People think it's haunted because it's next door to the crematorium. Sometimes it gets a bit smoky outside, but the room doesn't smell unless they are burning marijuana the police have seized."

The following day, we met the applicants. We interviewers sat in groups of three. I was assigned to work with a tall, meaty American statistician from the WHO, a man I always considered a jerk. Dodong Capul, the token Filipino from USAID, was there. He was a proud Cebuano and looked back to retiring back to Cebu, the California of the islands. I was among the many who wished for his retirement, too.

Dodong asked the first applicant if she would be willing to learn from an American. The young doctor looked at us with big brown eyes. "Yes. The materials said it was an American project, and we would learn to be like the American CDC."

Dodong stared hard as if trying to peer into her soul. "If you say so."

He asked each interviewee the same question and gave

each the fisheye. All swore they wouldn't mind, and they didn't. Over the years, nobody dropped out, let alone protest my being American. After I made extensive edits to their scientific papers or reports, a couple of trainees called me a white monkey without a tail, always in clear English to be sure I understood. Later, I realized Dodong was probably embarrassed about joining the arch-colonialist USAID and trying to establish his creds.

We took about two-thirds of the applicants and called it a day.

Budsy had spent this time hanging out with relatives and buying clothes and jewelry to sell when she returned. Her eyes shone with excitement. "I went to the embassy and picked out a house for us. I'll show you tomorrow."

It turned out to be a big airy tropical mansion in a place called Magallanes Village.

As Budsy showed me through the big rooms, she said, "I'll like being back home," she smiled, "as long as I live like a queen."

And she did.

CHAPTER 10
THE HAUNTED OFFICE

udsy stayed home the first week. Every morning, I hiked the half mile from our house to the LRT, the superb elevated light rail system that's the fastest way to get across the choked streets of Manila. Twenty minutes later, I stepped into the smoky streets of Tondo, crossed the road, entered the Department of Health (DOH) compound, and finally arrived at our haunted office by the crematorium.

On the first day, a couple of trainees from Mindanao—Bong Conanan and Simer Belacho—investigated the haunting. If you opened the front door quickly, the back door would open, and vice versa. Within two minutes, they found that the ghost was caused by air pressure: When one door opened, the air pushed the opposite door closed. Our first encounter with science had gone well.

Simer was from Mindanao, which was in a constant state of civil war with the Muslim National Liberation Front (MNLF), which occasionally overran towns and held them for weeks, but mostly they limited themselves to kidnapping people and holding them for huge ransoms.

Simer told me that American soldiers in Mindanao once used a helicopter with a heat sensor to trace a pizza truck traveling to a rebel stronghold and rescue a hostage. It sparked a massive kerfuffle over it being "an insult to national pride." The Americans had to leave.

"Of course, the police and army are splitting ransom money with the MNLF." Simer smiled ruefully. "It's in all their interests to keep the rest of us down."

"Doesn't the Manila government send much money for aid?" I asked.

"Some, but most of it goes to the richest few. We send far more money to Manila in taxes. That's why we call ourselves the cash cow of the country."

Another guy from the south was Willie Pastor, a chubby little character who lived on the little round island of Bohol. He came from a military family and claimed to be an army deep penetration agent in the MNLF. We learned later that he wove so many stories that you couldn't trust him.

Manolet gave the first lecture of the day and announced he would be teaching statistics and that I'd do the rest of the day. It wasn't a bad deal for me. He was busy assisting Dr. Bengzon, so it was no surprise that he couldn't teach every day. I often taught eight hours a day. Since the afternoons were dedicated to group problem-solving, it was doable.

Bebes Benabaye was a bright and dedicated young doctor from Cebu. A few years after she graduated, she became Regional Director for all the Visayas, the islands in the center of the country.

The afternoon case studies were fun. Trainees worked as a team to solve a problem I brought from CDC. It takes teams to stop epidemics, so it was critical our trainees learn to work in teams the way we did at CDC.

The course began smoothly, but about three weeks later, an army general led a coup attempt. I heard about it during the afternoon group problem. A sound like popcorn popping outside caught my attention. I assumed the crematorium was cooking up some dope the cops seized, but the sounds continued.

I asked someone to walk up to the board and calculate an odds ratio. No one spoke. I called on Willie. He stood and said, "We can't concentrate, Dr. White. The gunfire is making us jittery."

"That's gunfire?" I said.

They all looked at me.

"OK, class is dismissed until the coup is over. You may go home whenever you want."

I zipped out the front door, across the big street, and up into an LRT car for home. The coup attempt was over before evening.

A couple of days later, Willie told us that the general who led the coup attempt had left a computer with an encoded hard disk when he ran away. He claimed they gave it to him, but he couldn't crack it, so the police were forced to pay an expensive hacker to do it.

A week later, he said, "The general's in one of those love hotels every Wednesday and Saturday." Love hotels are expensive rent-by-the-hour places where men and their mistresses hook up. Not only are there mirrors on the ceilings, but also features like saltwater aquariums on the walls.

I tried to persuade Budsy to try one. "You think I'm a slut?" she growled. "I'm enough for you or any other lucky man. I don't need props and theatrics. I can make a man excited with a smile." And so she could.

They caught the coup leader in a love hotel a week later, as Willie predicted. Military justice treated him gently. They kept him under house arrest for a couple of weeks, then released him. I think this lenient attitude contributed to the many subsequent coup attempts. Interestingly, the troops involved in the coup mustered at McDonald's and Shakey's restaurants around Manila.

As Manolet's work with Dr. Bengzon took up more of his

time, I found myself teaching most of the time, no matter the subject.

I never seemed to have enough time to make up statistics examples, so I made them up as I talked and worked problems through in front of the class. Unfortunately, I'm lousy at arithmetic, so I often make mistakes. Filipinos are polite and respectful, but the trainees had to correct me, and they loved it. In a sense, my incompetence in math was a teaching tool. Everybody focused on catching me yet again.

Conky, the flamboyant lady from Tarlac, often did, and she corrected me with great pleasure and triumphant laughs.

One day, I began to get hoarse and cough.

Cecile Mañalac, our skinny nurse Filipina-Chinese administrator, took pity on me. "You need some salabat for that throat."

"What's salabat?"

"Ginger tea. I'll make some in your big cup."

Sure enough, the tea worked. I was well through my second lecture of the day when I felt a fuzzy buzzing between my lips. I spit out a giant fly.

Conky jumped out of her chair with delight. "He drank a *bangaw*." *Bangaws* are giant flies, the kind you find on rotting corpses out in the woods. Our building was next door to a crematorium. It didn't bear thinking about.

The class erupted. I reached down with as much dignity as possible, picked up the fly, and tossed it in the wastebasket. Conky put a graceful hand over her full lips to cover her laughter as everyone slowly quieted. Conky would look at one of the other women, and they would burst into giggles again.

I said, "It's not that funny."

"You're right," Bebes Benabaye choked out.

The class treated me with elaborate courtesy for the rest of the day. I only caught a few smiles in my peripheral vision. Still, they were trying to make me feel better.

Back in Magallanes Village, Budsy had been buying and selling jewelry. She got bored and started accompanying me to classes to hang out there. One day she stayed home and made brownies for the class. I passed them out at lunch.

Nobody seemed able to concentrate on the afternoon group case study, one of my favorites. That evening, Budsy asked how my day went.

I told her, and she laughed. "None of your trainees have ever had marijuana. They asked me to get some for them. My sister brought over a bag, and we made them nice strong brownies."

"If only I'd eaten one, I could have stopped it."

"But you didn't," she giggled. "My sister is going to have some new customers."

If word got out, this could wreck the whole program. If Dr. Bengzon found out, it could be an international incident. CDC would fire me for unethical behavior. I might not even be able to get my old job back in Flushing. I couldn't risk a repeat of her recklessness.

"Budsy, I'll have to send you back to the US. You're too big a risk."

She wept. Of course, I couldn't send her back.

Manolet saved us. We detected epidemics by reading the newspapers. By the time the reporters picked them up, hundreds of people might be sickened. Manolet offered Budsy a job organizing a sentinel surveillance system for infectious diseases so we could find and stop epidemics before they spread. She agreed to take on Manolet's wife's little brother, Oca. He was losing money driving a jeepney route and needed a job.

Oca barely spoke English, but he was a self-taught genius at fixing computers and broken data files.

Manolet and I gave Budsy a list of diseases prone to cause epidemics, then worked out how her weekly report would look. The obvious place to start was the famed San Lazaro

Hospital, the fever hospital conveniently located five minutes away from our offices in the same compound. Franciscan monks founded the hospital for lepers in 1598. Interestingly, it housed no lepers when I was there in the 1980s. In modern times, you can easily treat leprosy with pills, so you no longer need special hospitals. Those with extreme debilities went to remote Culion Island, off the vast and deeply forested Palawan Island. In the US, they went to scenic Molokai Island in Hawaii or the Carville Leprosarium in Louisiana. When I was an EIS officer assigned to Arkansas, I received my first and only official telegram from Carville, where they had discovered that you could grow leprosy in the footpads of armadillos. They wanted to learn whether leprosy bacilli could be found in wild armadillos in the US without stirring up public hysteria.

We organized the sanitarians, who typically inspect restaurants and water systems, as armadillo catchers. They invited me, but I foolishly missed the opportunity to tour the famous laboratory. I'm not sure if the hunt was like a holiday rodeo or if they put out traps. In any event, they caught a bunch of the rascals and drove them to Carville.

I only saw a few cases of leprosy in the Philippines. Once, Budsy's sleazy brother-in-law, Rene, brought in a pregnant woman with a nasty rash. He worked as a fixer in the Quezon City government and thought I might be able to help. She was maybe seven months pregnant. She had a rash on her nose and no sensation in her fingers or on her raised skin rash. I saw a red scar on two fingers, where she had burned them with a cigarette without noticing. Classic leprosy. *Mycobacterium leprae*, a cousin of the germ that causes tuberculosis, causes it.

M leprae prefers cool temperatures, so it likes to grow in the nerves on extremities like noses, fingers, and toes. A similar mechanism accounts for the pattern of black on Siamese cats. The cats are really black, but they have a temperature-sensitive gene mutation for albinism that only works on warm parts of their fur, so the cool parts remain black.

People dread catching leprosy, but it's rarely contagious.

Fear of leprosy led to the construction of San Lazaro back in the 1500s. It's named for Lazarus in the Bible.

On her first day as surveillance czar, Budsy made an appointment with the director, who agreed to cooperate with conditions: Budsy could never visit patients or nurses on the wards. She'd need to rely on the hospital nurses and go to the lab, but that was it.

She met with Manolet and me. "I need quality data, or my analysis will be useless. Maybe even misleading." Her eyes blazed, and she got up and paced. "This is my first job with the DOH, and I'm already about to fail." I could see sweat popping out on her forehead.

Manolet looked at her. "These are serious charges. I'll tell the secretary and see what steps he wants us to take."

ARAB, a superb manager, was quick to respond.

Manolet later told me, "He's ordered the director to allow you to collect whatever information you need. If she refuses, he'll fire her. You know how he hates corruption."

The next day, Budsy and her first surveillance nurse attacked San Lazaro and counted the patients in every ward. "There are six hundred ghost beds," she told us.

I asked, "What are ghost beds?"

"Imaginary beds that exist only in the books. The department pays each hospital by the bed, so more than half the money we send to SLH disappears with the administrators and their *kasabwat*."

"What's *kasabwat* mean?"

She sneered. "Crony. Coconspirator."

Manolet looked pained. "This is worse than we thought. Set up your site. I'll tell Dr. Bengzon."

A day later, Dr. Bengzon summoned me. "Mark, that place

is riven with crooks from top to bottom. I'm thinking of closing it."

"Sir, San Lazaro still serves a lot of people. I suggest you fire the top administrators and put in a new director, someone tough enough to clean it out.

The Secretary and Mario contacted the heads of major infectious disease programs. None had wanted to waste time cleaning the Augean Stables of SLH. They all thought we should close it and farm out the patients to their programs. I'd have said the same thing if I was in their place.

So Mario brought in Bio Gonzales—an endocrinologist, superb manager, tough guy, and diabetes specialist. A month later, Bio invited Budsy and me over.

"I heard about your great work," he said, offering us diabetic candies. "I'll handle the administration. I want your opinion on starting a diabetes and endocrine clinic."

"I can see a diabetes clinic, but I hope you'll keep the infectious disease beds." I paused. Obviously, he was going to do it, and I needed to persuade him to keep the infectious disease program.

"Of course. I want Budsy to take me on a tour to get to know the doctors and nurses on the floors."

"With pleasure," she said quickly.

I heard them chatting happily as I stepped out the door and headed back to DOH. Two weeks later, she wrote her first weekly report to Dr. Bengzon and a few dozen other people in DOH.

Soon, health reporters began asking for copies. Budsy had to be more careful about what she wrote, but the news reports led many mayors and governors to take action to fix water supplies and close down dirty restaurants.

The system was so successful that Budsy built a national network, and many other countries followed our example.

I visited San Lazaro often to examine interesting patients

and help the residents out. Soon, Bio introduced me to the chief resident, a big guy named Eric Tayag.

"Dr. White, I'd like to ask you to present at our Grand Rounds. About half the time, they present a patient where nobody is sure what's causing their symptoms. The other half, it's a patient where the doctors know the diagnosis but need ideas on how best to treat it. I asked other infectious diseases specialists to give Grand Rounds, but all refused. Will you join us?"

"You bet, Eric.

"See you next week," he smiled.

When I showed up for rounds, the big hospital auditorium was filled with white-coated doctors, students, and nurses. I'd seen the most challenging cases New York City could throw at me, so I was pretty confident.

The first week, they pitched me a classic case of systemic lupus erythematosus, a disease caused when you become allergic to your own body tissues. It produces high fevers and looks like an infection.

I discussed the diseases that might cause this picture, and the differential diagnoses, then summed up, "This looks like lupus, but it could be disseminated tuberculosis."

Silence.

Eric said, "You're right, Dr. White. How'd you do it?"

"You chose a disease that I frequently saw in the US. If you want to catch me, try tropical diseases."

People applauded loudly, and a few patted me on the back as I walked out. It felt great.

In subsequent weeks, I learned that they didn't do lumbar punctures to diagnose meningitis for fear of lawsuits if something went wrong. They'd never had a positive blood culture. When they got an autopsy, the pathologist just opened the patient up and looked inside. They said, "We don't see the need to do microscopic autopsies."

It became clear that in many cases, they presented me with

cases where they didn't know, then accepted my diagnosis as the answer. It worried me.

Eventually, I said something that hurt somebody's feelings, and Eric had to cancel my rounds. The training program for residents was teaching them the wrong way to practice medicine.

Manolet suggested I talk to Medy Saniel, director of the Research Institute for Tropical Medicine (RITM), the equivalent of the US National Institutes of Health (NIH). RITM was a world-class laboratory, and their many millions of dollars in grants came from the US NIH and other first-world equivalents.

Medy was a Waray from Samar, a fierce tribe. Budsy explained that the tribal anthem included *Manigas ka* or "We will stiffen your body," as in rigor mortis.

RITM's modern building complex sat outside Manila on a vast tract of land. When I entered Medy's office, I found that she was about Budsy's height with a no-nonsense hairdo and piercing black eyes. She was on the Field Epidemiology Training Program (FETP) board. The final exam was an epidemic report that each student had to write and defend. Medy terrified students—and a few board members, including me.

I knew she was suspicious of Americans, so I tried to impress her with my knowledge of the country. "I notice that the heads of most large institutions are women. So is the president. It seems you have a matriarchy."

"What's wrong with that?" she said, rising from her chair to look down at me across her desk.

We later became friends, and she urged me to emigrate, knowing I loved the people and country.

"We can't take on fixing the whole residency program, but we can train Eric. Then Bio can help Eric improve things."

She arranged for Eric to work for a few months as a RITM resident to see what a real research hospital looked like.

Medy showed me that I could be happy and productive in a matriarchy. Matriarchs like Medy are passionate about making life better for everybody, particularly the poor.

And matriarchs usually don't order armies to shoot people.

That was when Medy made me a feminist.

CHAPTER 11

THE MAN WHO KILLED MAGELLAN

One Sunday morning, I walked down to a breakfast of milkfish and rice and found Budsy at the table, sitting in front of a pile of opened newspapers. The headlines were variations of "Don't Eat Fish. It's Poisoned!"

No fish? People ate fish every day. Fish was cheap and available everywhere. Most of the protein in people's diets came from fish. If the poor couldn't afford meat, they were at risk of malnutrition.

"Looks like I'll be having eggs for breakfast."

"Don't be a baby," she said. "I already finished mine, and I feel fine."

Red tides had appeared off many islands, and people were getting paralyzed minutes after eating mussels.

Budsy pointed to an article in the *Manila Bulletin* and read, "Poisoning is caused by eating shellfish, but the Bureau of Fisheries and Aquatic Resources, BFAR, advises the public to be on the safe side and avoid fish as well."

"I'm surprised they didn't warn against beef and pork, too," Budsy sneered. The idiots at BFAR were causing a national crisis, basing decisions on "an excess of caution," which usually leads to problems.

Manolet called, and we drove into Manila to meet him in

the library and read up on PSP. When we arrived, he sat at a big table, books and medical journals heaped in front of him.

"Mark," he said, "BFAR called and said there's an epidemic of Paralytic Shellfish Poisoning (PSP) in Bataan."

I felt my body jump. Bataan is across the bay from Manila, home to nearly ten million people.

Manolet said, "I told BFAR you are my assistant and gave them your phone number."

"Thanks, piles."

"Better you than me. Do you know anything about red tides?"

"Nope. We have them in the US. I lived in the middle of the country, and we didn't eat a lot of shellfish."

He slid a thick textbook across the table. It said red tides are caused by tiny organisms called dinoflagellates. I skipped ahead to find the symptoms and treatment.

Budsy held up another book. "Do you know some people think dinoflagellates are plants? They argue with people who say they are animals." She smiled happily. She loved a good argument.

"They are considered algae because they can generate energy from sunlight using chemicals similar to chlorophyll. People say they are animals because they swim using tiny whiplike tails, flagella. Guess where the name came from?"

Manolet was bending over a thick volume. He reached his hand around his back like he was whipping himself. He said, "They don't make toxins all the time; only when they bloom."

"Bloom?" Budsy said, "Like flowers?"

Manolet said, "When there are lots of nutrients in the water, the population explodes and covers miles of ocean. That's the bloom. Sometimes pollution from cities seems to set them off. Other times ocean currents wash the nutrients in from out to sea. Maybe they make the toxins to kill off rivals."

None of the books mentioned anybody getting poisoned from eating fish. We learned that shellfish make their living filtering the water and eating the little animals and plants that stick to their gills. It was easy to see how they could concentrate the poison, which doesn't affect them.

PSP has a distinct clinical picture. You get sick a few minutes after eating the shellfish.

Victims of the neurological form of PSP usually describe numbness and tingling in the lips, mouth, and face within minutes of eating contaminated shellfish. They get weak and, in severe cases, can get paralyzed, so they can't walk. If the paralysis affects the respiratory muscles, they can die unless put on a respirator.

I knew something about the waters of Manila Bay because I used to take beer-soaked cruises around Manila Bay with Quasi Romualdez, Dean of the University of the Philippines Medical School. A dapper man with short, gray-white hair and a pencil mustache over his upper lip, he pointed out the huge pipes pouring brownish raw sewage into the water, launching armadas of plastic bags for miles. He once took a swallow of beer and told me, "Don't let anybody tell you that 'Dilution is the solution to pollution.' It ain't so."

There was plenty of food to make algae bloom in the bay.

Our outbreak was in the little town of Limay, Bataan. Bataan (pronounced "Bat-ah-an," not "baton") is on the mountainous peninsula where Filipino and American troops made their last stand against Japanese invaders in WWII. You could see the coast across the bay from Manila.

We loaded up our car with trainees. The team leader was Ilya Abellanosa. I once asked her if her parents named her after a Russian. She smiled and shook her head. "It means 'I love you always.'"

Her long, shiny black hair announced she was seeking a husband, and her beautiful black eyes inspired both love and fear. She had a sharp, sharp tongue—my kind of girl.

A couple of hours later, we arrived in Limay. Sunlight filtered through the dusty air. When we stopped to ask for directions, people peered at me, whispered, and pointed. *Not much happens here*, I thought.

In a few minutes, we reached the beachfront *barangay* where the outbreak began. *Barangay* is the name of the boat the Malays sailed in when they invaded the islands and kicked out the tribes living there before them. Now it means "neighborhood." A proud bit of history—if you're descended from the Malay tribes.

The *barangay* captain met us and showed us around. He was a thin man in an old T-shirt and shorts with a dapper white mustache. "People started getting numbness and tingling around their mouths, then they usually got dizzy, and their hands and feet got weak."

The captain said three people got short of breath, and two had to go to the hospital to get on breathing machines. "Two other guys died before we could get them to the hospital. Strong young men. People said they ate a lot of mussels."

Ilya asked if they'd eaten fish.

"Everybody eats fish," he said.

Ilya had brought questionnaires, and the trainees fanned out to survey the people to ask them what they'd eaten and if they'd gotten sick. They were back in two hours, and Ilya made tables so we could interpret the data.

"Every single person who got sick ate mussels," she said. "Some people who ate mussels didn't get sick, and nobody who only ate fish, vegetables, or rice got sick. It's the mussels."

Ilya's team had solved the outbreak.

"I'm proud of you all," I said. "Normally, we tell people what to do to avoid getting sick. Here, everybody knows already, so there's no need."

Ilya said, "Captain, we'll be sure you get copies of BFAR's weekly reports. They'll tell you when it's OK to eat shellfish again."

The captain was not happy. "Fish doesn't cause this disease, right?"

"Right," I said. "According to what we've read, fish never cause paralytic shellfish poisoning. That's why it's called shellfish poisoning."

The captain frowned. "We're fishermen here, but everybody is so scared that even our families won't eat fish. If we can't sell fish, people won't be able to survive."

"Wait a minute," Budsy said. "Remember the embalming fluid crisis?"

It was impossible to forget.

In the days after the Marcos dictatorship ended, nobody knew whom to trust. After decades of government lies, nobody believed anything the government said. As in the twenty-first century, conspiracy theories swept the country nearly every week. In the early days of the Aquino government, a rumor circulated in a small town that the fish in the market looked "too fresh." Someone got the idea that fish vendors were adding embalming fluid to the fish to keep them looking fresh, and others began to notice the same thing. When fishermen sold fish right off their boats, they also seemed too fresh. Many people concluded that the fishermen were in on it, too. Newspapers began to ask how long people had been eating embalming fluid.

The Japanese government had given the Philippines a beautiful food and drug laboratory (BFAD) with the latest precision instruments. BFAD's first win was when it tested an assortment of antibiotic pills and found several companies were selling sugar pills that didn't contain any antibiotics. Dr. Bengzon pulled them off the market and charged the owners with crimes.

People began submitting fish to test for formaldehyde, the active ingredient in embalming fluid. Any citizen could submit samples to BFAD and get a report in a few days. Most of the samples turned out negative, but a few showed two or three parts per billion of formaldehyde, the main ingredient in embalming fluid. More and more people sent samples, and BFAD found positives from all over the country.

People stopped eating fish, plunging the economy into a crisis. The poor fishermen were losing millions of dollars a day.

Concerned, we surveyed fish markets in Manila and asked Budsy's nurses to send samples from all over the country. Some were positive, but there was no pattern. We surveyed people who had eaten the positive fish, but nobody seemed to get sick. The DOH issued a press release with our preliminary findings. The newspapers had an answer. The formaldehyde probably was causing cancer. We just had to wait long enough, then thousands, maybe millions, of people would come down with cancer. It's nearly impossible to fight dedicated conspiracy theorists.

With no sick people, we were stumped. I didn't know what to do. Our method was to start with sick people, then work backward to see what made them sick. We had no tools to discover whether an exposure caused an unknown health risk. We called CDC in Atlanta and learned that it took years to decide whether a chemical in the diet put people at risk of disease. You needed teams of chemists, toxicologists, epidemiologists, and statisticians to work for years to find out. We did learn that the formaldehyde levels in our fish were millions of times less than the WHO allowed in food or water, as well as the standards set by CDC, EPA, and the US Department of Agriculture.

I called the toxicologists at CDC. A woman with a reedy voice picked up. "I see your problem," she said. "The WHO compiles this book of all the chemicals you find in foods. It's called the *Codex Alimentarius*. There are dozens, maybe hundreds of volumes. Check with your WHO office."

So Budsy and I headed across Manila to the WHO Regional Office. A pleasant guy with thick glasses showed me the books and helped me look up the most familiar species of fish Filipinos ate.

"You see, most fish contain a few millionths of a gram of formaldehyde. You know why, right?"

"Of course. Cells use the Krebs cycle to turn sugar into ATP, which cells can use for energy. Part of the cycle is formaldehyde."

"I'm impressed. You paid attention in biochemistry class."

"Not all doctors are idiots at chemistry."

He gave me a fishy stare and helped me make copies of the critical pages. Next, I brought these to the trainees. We wrote a report explaining why fish was safe to eat and that nobody had adulterated it. The response was headlines that included "DOH sells out to fish industry" and "National Conspiracy Risks Nation's Health."

While I'd been looking up the book on fish, Budsy had scanned through other volumes. Every food she found contained minute levels of formaldehyde, which is not surprising because every cell must make energy.

A team of trainees went to the Manila docks, hoping to interview some fishermen. A big yacht pulled in, and the Australian ambassador stepped off with a big bag of fish he'd caught. He was happy to help. The trainees called some health reporters and asked them to meet us at the Australian Embassy.

A reporter from the *Manila Chronicle* said, "With all due respect, we'd like to meet you at the docks." When they arrived, two reporters took the ambassador's bag of fish and climbed into the back of the ambassador's limousine with him. They never left it alone and even stood in the kitchen as the cooks made dinner.

The dining room was crowded with trainees and reporters as the ambassador bit into his first slice of fish. "Fresh and good," he proclaimed.

A reporter piped up. "How do we know you aren't lying to protect the fishermen?"

"Don't be daft! I don't live here. Do you think I'd risk Australia's good name for some grubby fishmongers?"

The reporters agreed he had no dog in this fight.

They remained unconvinced that the fish usually contained minute amounts of formaldehyde, so we drove in a caravan to BFAD with the reporters carrying some fish. The results showed the same tiny levels of formaldehyde that other samples had shown.

We invited the reporters to join us when we fried some of the fish we tested. Nobody came, but we'd convinced them because the headlines joined us in assuring people they could eat fish again.

The wave of hysteria evaporated.

Back in Limay, Budsy said, "So maybe we can get the Australian ambassador to come here and eat some more fish."

Ilya said, "You and Dr. White can eat the fish. If you don't get paralyzed, people will believe us!"

"What do you mean 'If I don't get paralyzed?'" I said. A frisson of anxiety tingled in my chest.

"Figure of speech," Ilya said.

I turned to the barangay captain, who was already leading a crowd of fishermen into town to make arrangements with the mayor. He looked back and waved before he disappeared down the street.

We found ourselves in the town's plaza an hour later, chatting with the mayor and the barangay captain. Fishermen set up metal barbecue grills and went to work. The fish smelled great. Street vendors sold peanuts and fruit. Somebody connected a boom box to a speaker system, and the music drew a crowd. Reporters and photographers stood around. There was even a TV camera. They put up a folding stage, and the mayor—a portly man with a mass of gray hair and big hands—climbed up, announced the plans for the evening, and stepped down. The barangay captain and a helper brought up a table and chair.

Only one chair. I was to be the only test animal. I looked at Budsy, but she was talking to Ilya. Neither offered to join me. Someone took my arm and led me to the stage where fishermen trooped up, each leaving a large plate on the table. The boombox began playing the kind of music you hear in a scary movie when the monster is about to grab the leading lady and tear her head off. I looked out at the happy people and wondered if the crowd at a hanging looked like this.

I lifted the fork and knife with heavy hands and took a bite out of a nice slice of grouper. The music stopped. Someone, I think Ilya, gasped.

Nothing happened. I took another bite. It was delicious. I realized I hadn't had lunch. I took one bite from each fish on the table for the next few minutes. I felt a little sweaty. There might have been a slight tingling around my mouth. I looked down at Budsy. She had a faint smile on her face. I worked my way down the list of symptoms until I reached the big one: breathing. I took a deep breath and coughed slightly, then burped. I said, *"Patawarin niyo ako,"* which means "excuse me."

Then I stood up, leaned over the edge of the stage, and asked for a napkin. The happy music started. Budsy and Ilya came up and sampled the fish. Soon the fishermen were serving the crowd, and we all had bags of fish to take home to Manila.

The barangay captain shook my hand. "I'd like to compliment you on your bravery."

"I knew I wouldn't get sick. It didn't take courage."

"Didn't anybody tell you that the NPA killed an American here this morning?"

"What?"

"They like to celebrate the anniversary of their founding

by killing an American. Usually, they get them in a McDonald's parking lot."

"Thanks for the warning," I said and slammed the car door.

After this, we handled all red tide outbreaks this way.

Red tide poisoning can come from any shellfish. We found it in scallops when we investigated an outbreak in Lapu-Lapu City on the island of Mactan. When the Spanish colonized the Philippines, Magellan got off his ship to battle the Cebuanos. Mactan's ruler, Chief Lapu-Lapu, killed Magellan with a stone axe. There's a massive statue of Lapu-Lapu with his axe on Mactan and many other places in the Philippines. The delicious national fish, grouper, is called *Lapu-Lapu*, after the chief.

Magellan's crew circumnavigated the globe, but not poor Magellan.

Only part of the city is on the main island. One barangay was on tiny Caubian island, about twelve miles of open sea from Mactan. Conky Lim-Quezon, Budsy, and I took a little outrigger to visit it. The sky was cloudy, and the waves rose with each mile until we slid back between waves, then surfed over the tops. The wind picked up, and I wondered if we might tip over.

Conky stood, both hands on the mast. Suddenly, she screamed, *"Pating, pating!"*

I looked at Budsy. She said, *"Patay* means dead."

"You mean Conky saw a dead fish?"

Conky's eyes were huge. She pointed. "Not a dead fish, a killer fish. It's a shark."

A big, black triangular fin traced a tight circle around us.

The boatman started a sharp turn, raising one outrigger above the water. I was holding on, but I felt myself sliding toward the water. I told the boatman, "Don't turn. It'll be better to go straight to the island. We're almost there anyway." My mouth was dry. I shivered.

The boatman yelled something at Budsy and sharpened the turn even more.

"Why is he still turning?"

She put her lips close to my ear. "He says he can't be responsible for killing a foreigner. If it were just us, he would have gone ahead."

Back on Mactan Island, I couldn't fall asleep, fearing I'd dream about being dismembered by a shark. The next day was clear, and we sailed to Caubian without trouble. The island had beautiful white sand, but the islanders had cut down all the trees for firewood, so there were no trees. It only took an hour or so to interview people and get samples of the scallops. When we were done, Conky asked a woman if she could use her bathroom. There were no bathrooms. The woman politely pointed with her lips to the sea.

The woman's husband brought Conky a burlap bag. "What am I supposed to do with this?" she said.

He put the bag over his head. The woman explained that this would keep her from being embarrassed. The rest of the islanders watched with interest.

Conky took the bag and wrapped it over her jeans like a skirt.

With a look of disgust, she walked slowly into the waves.

I'm sure they're still telling their grandchildren about the funny people from the mainland.

CHAPTER 12
BYE, BYE, MISS AMERICAN PIE

The US Embassy rented dozens of mansions, including ours, in the fancy Magallanes Village subdivision near Villamor Air Base during the Cold War, when communist guerrillas were viewed as the most significant threat. It never dawned on anybody that the military might be a greater menace.

But they were. Once, we woke sometime after midnight to popping noises like firecrackers. As the minutes passed, we wondered when the jokers with the firecrackers would stop. I went to the front door and stepped out into the velvety night. Night-blooming flowers' perfumes drifted lazily on the breeze. Usually, the sound of crickets, lizards, and nightbirds calling was almost deafening, but now it was only the popping-corn sound. It seemed to be coming closer and louder, then a sharp burst of noise to my left startled me.

Budsy appeared behind me, put a hand on my shoulder, and pulled me down into a crouch. We scuttled back through the door and slammed it behind us, reassured to hear the loud swoosh and bang of a heavy, well-hung door closing hard.

I looked at her face. "Was that guns? Do you think somebody was shooting at us with a machine gun?"

"Either that or an assault rifle on full auto."

"Thank God the embassy bought thick doors."

Budsy locked the door. "It's made of wood. It won't be much help if soldiers want to get in. Like if they want to take our money, kidnap you, or rape me." She glanced up the stairs toward the bedrooms. It was an ugly thought.

A fist of panic hit me in the stomach. Someone was shooting at us, perhaps communist rebels or even government soldiers in a military coup. My skin felt wet, and my knees trembled.

The embassy required us to take a security course, so we knew to go upstairs to the safe haven. This is a fortified room in your house where you can hole up if someone breaks in. The door is reinforced, and steel bars protect the windows. Ours was in our second-floor bedroom.

So we bounded up the stairs, side by side, hips and shoulders bumping. About halfway up, she elbowed me sharply. A smile crept across her lips. It was impossible not to smile back. We raced and giggled. We exploded into the bedroom together and fell on the bed. Budsy got up and slammed the heavy steel-reinforced door shut. She locked the two deadbolts, then launched herself at the bed and landed with an arm and a leg on top of me. Her eyes were bright, her smile broad as a full moon. She panted slightly and pressed her lips on my mouth so hard it felt like I'd been punched. Her body felt warm and sweet, like a bakery. As terrified as I was, my body responded. If you're frightened and in danger, making love feels like a good idea, at least for me. If things work out, you have a head start on repopulating.

"This isn't the time to be amorous," I mumbled into her mouth through our locked lips. Then I reconsidered. If we were about to die, why not?

I caught my breath and said, "Let's think back to the security courses at the embassy."

She said, "My favorite part was when they showed that

movie of the car blowing up with the fertilizer bomb. The way they talked about the ingredients, we could make one. Of course, we wouldn't do that unless we needed to."

She slid her warm skin against me. "I wish I had time to take the evasive driving course. I'd really like to learn how to hop the curb, up onto the sidewalk, and make a jug-handle turn."

The thought of Budsy's evasive driving was almost as terrifying as the rebels. To take the course, you had to bring your own car; ours was a low-slung sports car, a bright red Chrysler Laser. If she hopped the curb, she would tear the undercarriage out and leave the transmission and oil pan a tangled, smoking mess dragging on the road, showering sparks over the gas tank. The best evasive maneuver they taught was jug-handle turns. Moonshiners invented them to escape police on mountain roads. As the sheriff's car gets about fifty yards behind you, the driver suddenly pulls up on the parking brake and puts the car in a backward spin. If they do it right, they are suddenly facing the sheriff. The moonshiners floor it and force the sheriff off the road in a game of chicken. There was no doubt that my flamboyant wife would relish this.

She slid over me, arched back, and smiled down. I pulled her down tight against me. She dug her nails into the backs of my shoulders. Then a bullet thwacked into the wall just outside the window.

We made a quick inspection of the room. The windows weren't broken. If worse came to worse, we could seal ourselves into the bathroom. The door was smaller and heavily reinforced, making it harder to get through. We could hold out for days. We had plenty of water. I made a mental note to stash some food there next time we could get out.

Budsy turned on the emergency radio. It connected us— and everybody else—to the marine guards at the embassy.

The radio screeched like the collapsing metal must have sounded as the *Titanic* ground into the iceberg.

I turned down the volume, then followed the Xeroxed instructions taped to the radio. I was pleased and surprised to find the first channel worked. If somebody discovered our frequency and listened in, there was a list of channels to try.

A few seconds later, a voice said, "I think I can hear gunfire." Another chimed in, "There's somebody in the shrubbery. We need the marines to check it out."

A firm, irritated voice cut in. "This is the guard post. Keep the line free for emergencies. The more you talk, the more likely the bad guys will know our frequency."

"Can't you station somebody near the housing to protect us?"

"We have no credible reports that any of you are at risk," the clipped voice said. "Think about it. The purpose of the rebels is to overthrow the Philippine government, not to hurt Americans. These guys want us to help them put Marcos back." The marine ended his transmission with a loud click.

A scared child got on the radio and said, "They're shooting outside. I think they want to get into our house." You could hear shots in the background.

"Where are you?" The marine guard asked.

"Dasmariñas Village, near Fort Bonifacio." The kid was from an important family; only the very rich or top diplomats lived there. Unfortunately, this coup attempt had begun in Fort Bonifacio, a huge Philippine army base. The kid was close to the action.

"Can you come and get me?" He sniffed back tears, his high voice breaking. It sounded like he was twelve or thirteen years old.

The marine sounded distracted. "Hang on, son, all our people are tied up right now. Stay in your parent's bedroom with the door locked. Keep the radio on. Lie under the bed or on the floor under the window if a stray bullet comes in."

Sobbing, he said. "There are two windows on different sides of the room."

"OK, then lie on the floor by the bed on the side closer to the windows. Can you do that?"

"I guess."

"Call us if something bad happens, and we'll come and get you." The marine closed the connection.

I hoped the kid wasn't smart enough to realize that if somebody broke into the house, there was no way the marines could drive several miles through streets that might be blocked by fighting and rescue him. He knew, though. Of course, he knew.

"Well," Budsy said slowly, "now we know where we stand."

"Which is where?"

"We're on our own. The marines are stretched too thin to help. I can't see the police or security guards fighting the army."

"What do we do?" I asked.

"We'll think of something."

Following the safety instructions, we lay next to the bed. After a half hour, we climbed back up. If this were our last night, at least we would be comfortable before we went. We lay on the bed, eyes closed, streaming sweat, and drifting in and out of sleep. The embassy advised us against having lights on that might be seen from outside, but we eventually turned the lights on and tried to read.

Sometime before sunrise, the phone woke us. I must have fallen asleep and dropped the receiver as I reached for it. When I picked it up, a midlevel American diplomat's proud and helpful voice said, "Are you OK?"

"Fine, just dropped the phone."

"This is a message from the embassy," he said unnecessarily. "We want to inform you and other employees of the US government that it is our policy to support the Aquino government. There must be no question that we are encouraging the military rebels."

"Good to hear."

"Yes, we're showing our support and confidence in the Aquino government by stressing that we consider the coup essentially over. That may help her a little.

"All official Americans"—a category that included me, barely—"will go to work as usual. We're going to ignore the coup attempt."

"I'm a big supporter of President Aquino, too."

"Excellent. The usual vehicles will bring people to the embassy and the Roxas building."

"I work at the DOH in the middle of Tondo. Can you ask one of the drivers to take me?"

"Goodness, no. We're still on high alert. We need to be able to respond quickly if someone is in danger. Just take your usual route, and I'm sure you'll be fine." An edge of annoyance crept into his tone. He had others to call.

Budsy and I unsealed ourselves from our bedroom hideout and went down to breakfast. We turned on the TV and were distressed to see a dapper rebel military officer explaining that the rebels held most government buildings, including this TV station. He explained the soldiers were demanding a pay raise, which the civilian government refused to grant. The officers felt they had no choice but to replace the incompetent elected government until order could be restored.

Bastards!

The phone rang—at least the rebels were letting phone calls through.

My counterpart, Manolet, didn't say hello. "The rebels have put up a roadblock on the highway, and I can't get through. We need somebody in the office in case the media calls." He was in charge of media relations. "We must let

them know we're still there, that the department is still func-
tioning."

"I'll do my best."

"Good. I'll be in as soon as I can."

After this surreal conversation, my stomach clenched.
What had I agreed to do?

"Who was that?" Budsy said, poking a fork full of fish
at me.

"Manolet."

"You didn't just say you're going to work?" Her eyebrows
winked above her nose.

"I guess I did."

She laughed. "My hero. We'll pack you a nice lunch in
case you can't make it back and maybe some extra for
dinner."

"Thanks for the vote of confidence."

She saw me off, holding my attaché case in one hand and
lunch in the other. We walked together to the guard's gate at
the entrance. The guards looked skeptical but opened the gate
for me. After a few steps, I looked back. Budsy was standing,
hip-cocked, shading her eyes with a hand. She smiled.

I went to work on the speedy elevated train. The walk to
the LRT station seemed to last forever. I remember wondering
if somebody shot me, would they eat my lunch? Then I
turned the corner and faced three big tanks marked with the
Philippine flag. Then again, rebels probably wouldn't have
bothered to paint new markings. The only thing to do was to
stare straight ahead and ignore them, like in high school
when a gang of bullies walked toward you in the hall.

These were big bullies. I watched for one of the turrets to
rotate its big guns and zero in on me. I tried to walk close to
buildings I could dive into if they sprayed me with a machine
gun. I'd never been so scared in my life. I was so afraid I
forgot to piss my pants.

I walked unmolested between the enormous machines. They seemed to have the engines off. I remember thinking this must be a good sign. Then I was up the steps and into the station. A couple of minutes later, a train rolled up, like every other day. I got on, the only passenger, and we pulled out of the station. The song "American Pie" poured from the speakers over and over on a loop. Not clear what that meant, but it didn't seem good.

At the next six stops, only a few people got on. I stepped off the train at Tayuman Station in Tondo. It was a different world. Nobody seemed menaced or nervous. The hustle was the same. Nobody in the slum seemed to have heard a coup was on, or they didn't care.

I walked carefully across the avenue through the San Lazaro gates. The guards were gone. Maybe they had been transferred to some more critical government building. I doubted the DOH was high on anyone's priorities in trying to take over the government, so this made sense. I learned later the guards just hadn't shown up for work. Waiting to see who won, I guess.

The trainees were all there, nervously trying to study or chatting in low tones. Maybe they thought the rebels might hear them. I tried to give them a lecture, but it was hopeless. None of us could concentrate. We sent them home early. I headed for the LRT station. This time, three other people were waiting—a promising sign. Maybe things were returning to normal, or they might have been waiting for hours. A woman in blue jeans looked at me. She opened her mouth as if she might say something but was silent. An old man in a suit and tie said, "You're an American."

"Yes, I am." Maybe he was with the rebels looking to kidnap me. Why didn't I tell him I was a Canadian working for the WHO? That was the standard operating procedure. I guess I was too rattled.

"Things can't be too bad if Americans are out and about."

"I hope so."

Miraculously, a train arrived on time. I was relieved to hear they had stopped playing "American Pie" and announced stations, just like on regular days.

Back at my home stop, the tanks were gone. Budsy was waiting at the subdivision gate. Manolet called to tell me that the rebel barricades on the highway were gone and that he would be at work the next day. I reported there were no calls from the media. The government had taken back its TV station. It was now broadcasting soothing music and a loyal general who was asking troops to return to the barracks. He promised there would be no retaliation. Then they played the national anthem.

We only heard a few shots in our neighborhood for the rest of the day. The Philippines' biggest air base was just across the wall, and the rebels wanted it to surrender. So far, the doughty airmen were holding out. On the other hand, they weren't strafing or bombing the rebels, either.

By the following day, the government had broken the coup attempt. The Aquino government forgave them, including the general who had led it, Gringo Honasan. It turned out that he had drained the soldiers' retirement account to pay for the coup. So much for the soldiers' pay raise.

Unfortunately, the generals had a different playbook than President Aquino and her kitchen cabinet of pacifist nuns. Over the next few years, the generals viewed her mercy as a sign of weakness and launched a series of attempts to destabilize the government, then take over in a coup d'état. The soldiers mostly fired over each other's heads, so few were killed. They didn't have a dog in the fight between the generals and civilian politicians, and they didn't want to hurt anybody. However, they typically killed about three hundred people, mostly civilians, when the bullets they shot in the air fell back to earth on distant victims. Occasionally, a jumpy soldier would shoot somebody who confronted them.

Later coup attempts sometimes lasted for days. I would sit at home and try to read, listen to music, or do emails. We were jangled and snapped at each other. We ran out of beer once. "Budsy," I said, "we need to send the cook out for beer."

"The cook's at the wet market buying fish for dinner."

Budsy's niece and nephew lived with us, so I said, "What about the kids?"

"They're at the college in classes."

"Buds, I've got the coup jitters. I'd get it, but the embassy says Americans should stay in their houses."

"You drink too much anyway. I'm tired of you lying around like a big white worm. If you want it, you get it. I certainly won't."

So I stepped out into the afternoon. The rainy season was coming, and sunlight beamed through the clouds and green leaves, giving everything a bright, Kodachrome look. I didn't hear or see a single bird, and the whole way to the gate, I saw no one. The guards gave me knowing glances as if they knew I was doing something wrong. Were they under orders to report to the embassy that I went out? What if one was a rebel sympathizer who would call and let his friends know where to kidnap me? What if, what if, what if?

The street contained a smattering of people, apparently going about their business. Suddenly,

Finally, I reached the corner grocery store. A little bell on the door jingled. I tried not to jump. The man behind the counter stared at me with interest. I had this odd feeling that a rivulet of sweat would run down my temple and show him how nervous I was.

In the middle of the floor stood a stack of six-packs of San Miguel beer. Budsy said San Miguel was the patron saint of drinkers, but her knowledge of theology was nearly as sketchy as mine. I had made it this far and felt a bit of pride in breaking the rules and venturing into the potentially dangerous streets, and I decided to celebrate by getting a six-pack of dark beer. So, I picked up one six-pack of regular beer and another of Cerveza Negra and placed them on the counter. The grocer smiled, then turned away. He seemed to be laughing. I took out my wallet and handed him a five-hundred-peso bill. He stifled a laugh, said something in Tagalog I didn't understand, and gave me my change. A man behind me said, "Cerveza Negra is what women drink for menstrual cramps." I considered telling him my wife needed it, but I took the beer and walked out into the welcome anonymity of the street.

The embassy called at five the following morning and told us that Americans were to go immediately to a downtown hotel, where it would be easier to protect us. We quickly loaded the car and glided slowly out of the village, joining a slow procession of other Americans' cars. Our Filipino neighbors stood in their front yards and watched us silently drift past. We were like rats leaving a sinking ship. So much for standing with President Aquino.

We took Roxas Boulevard, one of Manila's biggest streets. It snaked along the shore and past the embassy on the way downtown. There was no sign of fighting. The usual traffic snarls seemed somewhat improved. It may have been the early hour. Then a giant American rode a big, black Harley past our column. He must have taken off the muffler because the bike bratted and snorted as he moved ahead like a motorcycle cop. When he reached the first car, he pulled up and knocked his fist on the window as if he planned to give the driver a lecture. He opened his mouth for the opening salvo. A big, ugly revolver appeared in the driver's hand. The biker left rubber as he shot ahead, winding through the traffic. Yet more unnerving weirdness.

Eventually, we arrived at the hotel. A crowd of Americans waited in their cars in a long, unruly queue snaking several blocks around a plaza swarming with people. Budsy sat behind the wheel and kept the motor running while I got out and stepped into the crowd of Americans milling about. I found my supervisor from USAID, who looked lost and unmoored. He seemed to be transforming from an executive to a refugee—his life in the hands of strangers. I asked him, "What's going on, Ken?"

"The plan is to stay in the hotel until they can fly us back to Washington. That way, the marines can protect us. Like circling the wagons, I guess."

"Doesn't that make it easier for the rebels to round us up?"

Fear flitted in his eyes. His voice quavered. "I agree, but we've got to follow the plan."

I learned a lot about coups and revolutions from Jimmy Hoover, who described himself as an ex–Army Ranger and visited us every six months. He was a doctor who worked somewhere in the US government. His muscles were hard and stringy, and the skin on his face was thickened and a bit red.

He took Budsy and me for beer-soaked dinners and told us stories about Americans escaping from unstable governments at the last second.

"I spent a couple of tours in Vietnam," he said and clinked his mug against Budsy's. "Getting the civilians out was a nightmare."

"It must have been a nightmare for the civilians, too."

"No doubt." He drank, his Adam's apple bouncing up and down.

"I was in Indonesia when the military took over in 1965. They were brutal. Killed the civilian leaders, hacked them up, and threw them into a well. No common sense. It was months before they could clear the bodies and decontaminate the well. Totally unnecessary.

"We had to evacuate in a hurry. People were shooting out their windows into the street. They didn't want to hurt us, just letting off steam. Had some tough times in Thailand, too."

It was hard to tell how many of his stories were true and how many were exaggerations or tall tales. He seemed to tease and test our credulity sometimes.

Jimmy reached into his bowl of goat stew and pulled out a chunk of meat and bone. "There's a pattern. Coups are short, almost always less than three weeks, usually two." He waved his goat bone to illustrate the point.

"The worst thing that can happen is if the State Department decides to evacuate Americans. They fly you back to DC and put you in a hotel somewhere in Northern Virginia."

"What's so bad about that?"

"Everybody in DC is covering their asses. It's a risk for these bureaucrats to take a chance on sending you back. If they do it too early and have to evacuate you again, it costs millions of dollars, and they can kiss their careers goodbye." He delicately placed his gnawed bone on the edge of his plate.

"They often keep you cooling your heels for six weeks or more."

"What other choice do we have?"

"I know some people in Indonesia, and I told them to expect you if there's trouble here. All you have to do is walk up to the Garuda, the Indonesian national airline, desk at the airport and tell them who you are and that you're my friends. They'll put you up in Jakarta until we know which way the wind is blowing. It'll be a lot less than six weeks."

"Won't we get in trouble with the embassy here?"

"They probably won't miss you until it's too late."

Following Jimmy's advice, I told Ken we would stay with Budsy's relatives and keep in touch. His boss came up and gave him some orders. They were so busy talking about the coup that I walked away without being forbidden to leave.

I headed quickly back to Budsy and hopped into the car.

"Let's blow this pop stand," she said and nosed out of the traffic jam, plotting a course toward our offices in San Lazaro.

No security guards were stationed in front of the department. No surprise there. Everything was humming along normally when we arrived and went to work. Staying the night wouldn't be a burden because we had couches in our offices.

One of Budsy's nurses ushered in some skinny, sweaty people at about six in the evening. They carried bags of food and drinks. I couldn't understand most of their Tagalog, but Budsy told me the guards rented them space to sleep in our offices at night. They were very humble and polite. It turned out the food was for our dinner.

In two days, the coup attempt ended. As usual, all the soldiers were pardoned, and the generals escaped.

There would be five or six more coup attempts.

We never got used to them.

CHAPTER 13
THE SANDWICH EFFECT

My two sons, Alex and Daniel, ages eleven and nine, respectively, spent a month of their summer vacation with us in Manila each year. One afternoon, Budsy and I took them to the US Embassy's Seafront Compound swimming pool. It was a perfect sunny afternoon. We were alone at the pool.

Both boys were skinny, blond, and pale, a gift from their German ancestors. I gave Alex a watch for his birthday, and he wore it in the water.

"Alex, take off your watch. You'll get it wet."

"No, Dad. It says it's waterproof."

"Your choice," I said.

Budsy and I sat in beach chairs, enjoying the light breeze, the kind Filipinos call *masarap na hangin*, or "delicious wind." We were alone beneath the bright-yellow sun and could've been in a travel poster.

Then I felt the earth sway a little beneath me. Small tremors are common in the Philippines, so I wasn't disturbed. The boys didn't seem to notice at all. Then the shaking increased. A power line sagged dangerously toward the pool; if it fell in the water, they might be electrocuted.

Water sloshed in a tidal wave out of the pool, along with

the boys and their toys. They stood and jumped up and down in delight. The shaking increased. Budsy and I jumped up from our seats and hurried, legs apart, to get them away from the shaking pool. We snatched up the kids and carried them to a clear area away from buildings, trees, and utility poles.

It was silent for about a minute when the shaking faded away. No buildings had fallen, then we heard a cacophony of horns from Roxas Boulevard, a few yards away.

We had arrived on the elevated LRT, so we walked the two blocks to the station to ride it home. When we reached the top of the stairs, the train sat next to the track as if some giant had picked it up and moved it. Derailed. Our house was about five miles away, so hiking would be difficult, particularly for little Daniel. We climbed back down and walked toward Roxas Boulevard. Everything seemed normal until Budsy flagged down a taxi. "That'll be twenty US dollars," the driver said.

She shrieked. "It should cost seven. There's been an earthquake. How can you screw the victims?"

The driver took a drink of some brown liquid and spilled some on his T-shirt. "It's capitalism, missus. I have to charge what the market will bear."

"You bastard," she said. There followed five tense minutes of negotiating. At one point, Budsy jumped up and down in a screaming rage. They settled on twelve dollars.

A few trees had fallen in our neighborhood, but the power lines and houses were OK, including our own. We settled down for an early dinner.

As I got up for a beer, the phone rang. It was Howie Severino, a reporter, and a good friend. He said, "The epicenter of the quake was in Baguio." Baguio City is nestled high in the mountains north of Manila. It's a famous tourist destination because it's cool year-round.

Howie took a breath. "The Hyatt there collapsed. Hundreds are dead. Landslides and huge boulders are blocking the roads into the mountains. The phone lines are dead. Baguio's cut off." He spoke in that urgent, breathless tone reporters use. "You've got to get me on a helicopter."

"Jesus, Howie. That's terrible. The Department of Health doesn't have a helicopter, and if it did, we'd need to send doctors and emergency medical supplies first."

"OK," he said, dismissing me. He hung up. The following day, his story was the entire front page of his paper, the *Manila Chronicle*, including a big picture of the devastation and an enormous headline: "Misery in Baguio. First Quake, Then Cold Rain." Howie later told me he and his photographer drove up the mountain roads, then walked over the big landslides and into town. After he got his story, he hired another cab to take him back to the landslide where he'd parked his car. Earthquakes are great times for taxi drivers.

Budsy and I drove to the DOH the next day. There had been an earthquake in Mexico a month earlier, so I emailed Dr. Ruiz, head of the Mexico FETP, for advice. A half hour later, he sent us a fax outlining what had happened and what he and his trainees had done. He described the survivors' psychological stages, which were similar to the Kübler-Ross stages of dying. First came relief that you had been spared, then guilt over surviving when friends and relatives had been crushed. Then came fear of aftershocks, irrational anger that authorities hadn't prevented the earthquake, and rage at the doctors and relief workers. Finally, they sank into depression. We made copies, then Budsy and I carried them to all the major offices in the department. It turned out that everything Dr. Ruiz said came to pass.

The following day, Manolet and I chose Conchy Roces, our fiercest trainee, to lead the team. Small and intense, she was passionate, with bright brown eyes and sharp intelligence. Conchy followed the truth relentlessly and never pulled her punches. She was a scion of an old Spanish-Filipino family of the generation that people said "spoke in Spanish to God, in

English to the press, and in Tagalog to their servants." Her father had been editor of the *Manila Times* when Marcos took over. When he and his bullies forced Conchy's father out of business, Conchy had to hold the family together as she served her pediatrics residency. People said she eventually joined the political opposition somewhere in the mountains, perhaps near Baguio.

Her assistant was Ivy Lopez, who was from the small town of Moncada. The trainees called her *Mutya ng Moncada*, the Pearl of Moncada.

Manolet and I went to Mario Taguiwalo, Deputy Secretary of Health. He said, "It sounds pretty bad up there. The president appointed me to coordinate the aid efforts, so I'll be moving there soon. Your team needs to get in first." He called the army, and they agreed to take Conchy and Ivy on a military helicopter. They took a change of clothes, a ream of yellow legal paper, and two heavy portable computers and headed to the air base. This was a terrible mistake—the first and only time we sent trainees into danger without accompanying them and sharing the risk.

Considering that no phone service was available in Baguio, we didn't know what was happening. Two days later, the road opened, and Budsy and I drove up. Most buildings looked OK, but occasionally, one was reduced to a heap of rubble. People wandered in a daze through the streets. We found Conchy and Ivy in the Provincial Health Office (PHO), putting together the results of surveys by making tallies on the yellow sheets. The yellow pads were the only useful things they brought.

Both women stood staring at us. When I asked what happened, Conchy began talking. "The helicopter took us to the big sports stadium because the airport was broken up and strewn with boulders. A crowd gathered below. They cheered. As soon as we landed, the people pressed in so hard we could barely get the doors open to get out. Then they saw we weren't bringing food, and the pushing stopped. The helicopter lifted off, and the next thing we knew, we were alone with all these hungry people.

"We stood there with our backpacks, the computers, and the box full of paper. For a minute, we thought the crowd would turn ugly, but in the end, they walked away, and we started to carry everything to the PHO ourselves. Finally, some guys helped us."

Ivy stared intently at me. It was difficult to avoid locking eyes with her. Her lovely black hair hung in strands down her neck.

The ground shook. People screamed and ran out into the street. Budsy and I nearly fell. Conchy, standing with her legs apart, endured the shaking with ease. "Some of these aftershocks are almost as big as the earthquake. People sleep outside in the rain rather than take the chance of being crushed.

"People don't want doctors; they want civil engineers to tell them if it's safe to move back inside and how to shore up walls."

Budsy put an arm on Conchy's shoulder. "Where are you sleeping?"

"In Roy Gavino's cousin's house. It's made of wood. Wooden houses rarely collapse in earthquakes."

Budsy waited a pregnant moment. "Is there room for us?"

"Of course."

Ivy stood, arms slack at her sides, looking at me. Just looking. I said, "Are you OK, Ivy?"

Budsy softly grabbed my arm. "I need to talk to you for a minute." When we were about twenty feet away, she said, "When a woman in the Philippines is furious with you, she won't talk to you. It's no use trying. Talk to Conchy if you need to communicate with her."

Conchy looked up at the cloudy sky. "It's getting late. There'll be rain soon. Let's walk to Roy's cousin's house."

"How far is it?" Budsy asked.

"A couple of miles, including detours around some streets blocked with wreckage." Conchy led the way, and I walked with her.

"You let us down," Conchy said. "Those computers are heavy, and there's no electricity, so they are worse than useless. We only brought one change of clothes, and we worked outside in the rain. Nobody in the health department here knew we were coming. Worst of all, we didn't bring food, and there isn't any here. Instead of helping the hungry homeless, we are the hungry homeless, just two more mouths to feed."

"Conchy, you're getting enough to eat now, aren't you?" I said.

"No. It's been especially hard on Ivy. We eat one meal a day, mostly a sandwich and a bag of juice."

"I'm sorry, Conchy. We'll do that next time."

"Next time? I hope to heaven there isn't a next time."

"Sorry, poor choice of words."

Ever since we arrived, we noticed the faint, nasty, cloying smell of rotting flesh around us. Now it was worse. Budsy looked at Conchy. "I'm surprised you can eat anything with this terrible smell." She scowled. "It's getting into my clothes and hair. I hope there's water we can wash in."

"There is. Roy's cousin has some rain barrels. It rains every day, so they're full.

"It smells so bad here because we're taking a detour to see the Hyatt Baguio. It was built to reflect the shape of the famous rice terraces on the mountainsides. The hotel is—was—built with floors like giant steps down the mountainside. When the quake hit, the hotel went down like a row of dominos. It must have been fast. I hope so. I'd hate to think of the people inside suffering."

"Are there still people trapped?"

"A lot of dead ones. That's why it smells so awful. A few

might be still alive, maybe stuck in little caves and airspaces made when the buildings went down."

We arrived at the mountainside where the hotel had collapsed. A few people stood around, staring aimlessly, hair slicked by the rain, clothes hanging. Each step of the building was about four stories tall. Bright white sheets tied together into long ropes hung down from windows, with each marked where somebody had escaped to safety.

It looked like they'd been laundered and were hanging out to dry. Everything, including us, was soaking wet and cold.

Conchy led us closer. Clouds of flies flew in and out of the wreckage, buzzing constantly. If you were stuck somewhere down in the rubble, the flies would drive you insane in half an hour. I opened my mouth to shout into the wreckage, hoping to find someone trapped. Then I realized how pointless that would be. Rescue teams would have been here long ago and probably revisited every few hours.

Conchy led us away, and we headed to the suburbs and Roy's cousin's house.

Roy Gavino was a big, strong guy—a malaria specialist. He brought food and supplies. He hadn't been on Conchy's misery tour, so he was in a celebratory mood. He brought several cases of beer, and his cousins said they had bought dog meat to make pulutan, a kind of food only men eat with beer. The dog meat made pretty good barbecue, particularly with Roy's special vinegar sauce.

Roy's cousin offered us his bed, but Budsy and I slept on the floor near the front door with everybody else. An aftershock woke everybody up every few hours, but we only ran outside once.

The following day, we met Mario, who was coordinating disaster relief from the PHO. He sat behind a wooden desk, the surface clear except for a cup of coffee and a roll. He was reading a newspaper, the *Manila Chronicle*, Howie's paper.

"Budsy and Mark! You've joined Conchy and me up here at last. I can't tell you how useful her surveys have been. There don't seem to be many injured people to help."

Surprised, I said, "But there must have been crush injuries when the walls came down."

"The first day, there were terrible injuries, big ones. They couldn't do major surgery on many people here because hospitals collapsed. A lot of the victims went into kidney failure and needed dialysis. I don't understand why."

At last, I could be helpful. "When something heavy falls on you, it crushes the muscles, which release the protein myoglobin into the bloodstream. It blocks your kidneys, and you may die in a few days unless you get hemodialysis, which permanently can cure your kidneys."

Mario leaned forward and said, "The first two days, US Navy helicopters took injured people to Manila for surgery and hemodialysis. You know, Larry Henares wrote in the *Manila Bulletin* that several anti-American politicians said things like, "I never thought I'd say this, but 'God Bless the United States.'"

Mario pushed himself away from his desk and smiled at us. "Look, I'm charged with managing the disaster, and I need information to decide what supplies to get and where to deliver them. A barangay captain just visited and said many of his people were going hungry. There must be dozens of other groups out there who need our help. Your job is to find them and let me know what they need. I'll expect your first report at five o'clock this afternoon."

So we headed out in the cold rain to find people who needed help. Budsy started at the edge of the city, then drove in spirals toward the city center the way you do in immunization surveys. When she came to a knot of people, she'd stop and we'd climb out, holding legal pads under our borrowed umbrellas. Usually, someone walked to meet us. We took these to be leaders and asked them what they needed. A typical interview went like this:

Conchy: "We're from the Department of Health, and we're here to see what you need."

Leader: "We need medicines. Lots of medicines."

Conchy: "Is somebody sick? What kind of medicines do you need?"

Leader: "Well, people have headaches, so we need something for that."

Conchy: "Any diabetics need insulin or people on high-blood pressure drugs?"

Leader: "I don't know. Just give us medicines."

Budsy: "How many people are in your group?"

Leader: "About a hundred and fifty."

Budsy: "We're just making counts. We don't have anything to give you."

Leader (looking surprised): "There are about twenty people left in the barangay. The rest went to stay with relatives."

The top requests were for tents and blankets, followed by food. Mario went to work on getting the stuff to the people we identified in the surveys, and things improved for the victims.

Even the people who had houses were afraid they had been weakened and might collapse in aftershocks. Everybody wanted structural engineers.

Conchy took us to the hospital to show us the surveillance system she and Ivy had set up. Two of Budsy's nurses waited with tally sheets for early signs of epidemics. No patients were waiting. The nurses said there were a few people on the second day, but only two since.

In disasters like earthquakes or volcanic eruptions, deaths and injuries happen immediately, but few health problems surface afterward unless there's an epidemic or starvation. Wars and famines are long-term disasters in which injuries, illnesses, and deaths continue to occur. Baguio had no epidemics, probably because of the rapid, effective government response.

Neighbors rescue most people injured in earthquakes long before rescue teams can come. Those pinned in the rubble after a day or two almost always die. Rich countries, including the US, sent big teams with sniffer dogs and heavy equipment to dig out victims, but they'd arrived several days late. Many of the team members wandered around, looking for ways to be helpful. Mario charged me with finding something for them to do. Measles immunization rates were low, so we organized them into teams and led them into the countryside, where they happily vaccinated away and probably saved some lives. Most of the millions of dollars that rich countries spent looking through the rubble for the last survivors could have provided tents, food, and blankets or rebuilt houses, hospitals, and schools. UNICEF was an exception. They set up big water tanks near the evacuees to provide clean water to drink.

Our survey results pointed to some hypotheses (theories) about why people were injured or killed. Next, we conducted a case-control study to determine how likely our theoretical risk factors accounted for death and injury. It was cold, slogging work.

Conchy, Budsy, and I spent several days hiking through the devastated city. All too often, the interviews went like this:

Conchy: "Do you know anyone who was killed or injured in the earthquake?"

Victim: "Yes, my uncle was killed."

Conchy: "Do you know where he was when the earthquake struck?"

Victim: "At work."

Conchy: "Do you know the kind of building and what he did after the quake hit?"

Victim: "No."

It was a real challenge, but eventually, even in the rain and with the aftershocks, we entered the data into Conchy's computer, which worked now that the electricity was back. We discovered the famous (to earthquake experts) sandwich effect. People on the bottom floor usually could run out before the building crumbled, so they survived. Tall buildings usually collapsed straight down, so the people on the top floor weren't crushed, either. But God help the people in the middle. They were at the greatest risk of being killed.

Conchy and the team published this as an article in the *Bulletin of the World Health Organization*.

A week after we returned to Manila, Manny Voulgerapoulis, head of Health and Population at USAID, told me we had been summoned to see the ambassador, the redoubtable Nicholas Platt. A career diplomat, he was, by all accounts, a good man.

In my two years in the Philippines, I'd never been invited to the embassy, which suited me fine. I was a scruffy field type, uncomfortable in a suit making small talk with "dips," as diplomats call themselves. Had they known of my existence, I'm sure they wouldn't have invited me—a marriage made in heaven.

Ambassador Platt occupied a big room with floor-to-ceiling windows looking out over Manila Bay. He rose and shook our hands. "Dr. White, I apologize for not inviting you to the embassy earlier, but you are here now. What can you tell us about the success of our aid to the earthquake victims?"

"Well, sir, the Filipinos were most impressed by the navy helicopters that took people with crush injuries to Manila. Ambulances distributed them to hospitals with hemodialysis units."

Manny said, "That was the navy. What about the rescue teams?"

I took a deep breath. "They arrived days after neighbors and Filipino teams rescued most survivors. They spent a lot of effort and money and found a handful of survivors. Next time, they could do more good helping evacuees and starting the rebuilding effort."

Ambassador Platt said, "The helicopters landed on the embassy roof. That helped, I'm sure." It certainly did. I realized the ambassador needed to justify his budget to the bureaucrats in Washington who divvied up the aid money. Just like me.

A few months later, the embassy staff invited Budsy and me to their Christmas party. After the party, we had to pass through the security gate. The guard closed the spiked iron door on our car at the entrance. I sat in the passenger seat, watching the spikes approach me and poke holes in the car door. "Floor it, Budsy. It's going to stab me!"

"No, it'll wreck the door."

It was like a James Bond movie where the bad guy puts Bond into an infernal machine. "Move it, damn it." She didn't.

The next day, we went back to the embassy and called the Regional Security Office to complain.

"You're the second car they've wrecked this month. The administrators say our policy is to pay Filipino employees minimum wage, so I can only get dumb ones. I've spent far more for repairs than we would have had to pay to increase wages enough to hire competent guards."

I don't know whether he got his new guards because the embassy never invited us again.

A perfect ending for all concerned.

CHAPTER 14
DANCING ON DYNAMITE

arthquakes can happen anytime, but Filipinos bring in the New Year like the Chinese, with tons of fireworks of every size and description. People shot off the usual assortment of firecrackers, rockets, Roman candles, and some exciting varieties I'd never seen.

Sinturon ni Judas (Judas' belt) is a long string of medium-sized firecrackers that squirm like fiery snakes when you light them and toss them on the ground. You have to be careful not to throw them on someone's leg.

Budsy showed me what looked like a matchbox. "These are *watusis*. Kids love 'em." She poured what looked like little pills on the sidewalk. "You can set them off by walking on them. Kids dance on them." I stepped on some. They snapped, crackled, and popped. I could see little flashes.

She said, "People say they're safe for little children because they barely explode, but they are tiny chips of TNT, fatal if kids eat them. A few children die from them every year."

Nonetheless, shooting off fireworks was great fun. My favorite was the chicken sandwich, a paper sandwich bag filled with gunpowder. A fuse stuck out of the opening like an aerial. You lit one of these babies, and the ground shook. I'm not kidding. They were invented after WWII when people dug up unexploded bombs and shells, carefully unscrewed them, and dipped out the gunpowder.

If all this sounds dangerous, it was. The government passed a law forbidding anybody to make or use them long ago. Fireworks companies went underground and soon increased production. Every year, they competed by making bigger, more dangerous explosives. They paid off the cops, who, like everybody else, spent New Year's Eve setting off fireworks themselves. People said, "You can't change our culture."

Every New Year's Eve, Rhais Gamboa, DOH's Undersecretary for Financial and Management Services, threw a terrific party. Budsy and I never missed it.

Rhais' parties started around sundown and ran very late. The first year, Rhais met us at the door, handed me a beer, and led us to the back lawn. DOH top management was all there, except Dr. Bengzon, who did not indulge in such silliness as New Year's Eve parties.

Mario Taguiwalo, the actor-turned-undersecretary, walked up to me with an egg.

"It's *balut*," he said.

"What's that?"

Budsy laughed. "It's a fertilized duck egg with the baby duck in it. They are supposed to make you smart. We used to eat them before we took exams."

Budsy cracked the egg on my head, then carefully peeled away the top half of the shell. "Open up and down the hatch."

She poured the egg into my mouth. I felt wet feathers sliding down my throat and stifled a gag.

We drank and ate *merienda*, delicious hors d'oeuvres, and told stories until midnight. We then drove home carefully, as many drunks were on the road, and people celebrated by shooting guns into the air, not considering that the bullets would come down somewhere. In a typical year, a couple of babies got killed when falling bullets hit them. Every New Year's Day, the US Embassy counted the spent bullets that fell on their roof. Usually, they found about three hundred.

In the first week of January, Budsy and her nurses noticed a sharp increase in tetanus cases at San Lazaro. The cause was clear. Many had lost fingers or hands from fireworks explosions. The wounds were filthy. The explosions drove dirt, paper, and swarms of tetanus bacteria into the skin.

Clostridium tetani, the germ that causes tetanus, makes a toxin that causes severe muscle spasms all over the body. Patients arch and twist into painful muscular seizures. Many can't swallow and die when stomach acid flows into their lungs. They get high fevers, abnormal heart rhythms, soaring blood pressure, and other nasty things. The heartbreaking thing is that you can prevent it by getting a diphtheria-tetanus-pertussis (DTP) vaccine during childhood or a tetanus vaccine as an adult. Cases rose every week through that January, then trailed off. Dr. Bengzon called Budsy to his office and told her to figure out how to prevent the epidemic the following year.

Manolet called a meeting, and we discussed what to do. "The problem here is the fireworks injuries," he said. "The first thing is that we need to get a better picture of who's getting injured and what they were doing when they were injured."

Budsy shifted in her chair. "That's easier said than done. Over a third of the patients died, and most of the rest went home."

"Let's make a team of trainees and nurses and do a survey to gather all the information we can," Manolet said.

We found little beyond what the National Epidemic

Sentinel Surveillance (NESS) system told us. It provided a telling description of the injuries, the most common being fingers or hands blown off. The awful medical word for torn-off flesh is "avulsed," as in, "The left hand was avulsed and traumatically amputated." Most of the injured and dead were young males, which made sense because young males shoot off the most fireworks. The ones with the worst tetanus had the most significant wounds.

However, the descriptive data didn't help us learn what people were doing that put them at risk for injury and infection. That required a kind of analytic research design called a case-control study. The idea is to examine the people who were injured or killed. These were the cases. We developed theories about what might have caused injuries. For instance, cases were more likely to shoot off big fireworks than those who did not. The controls were neighbors of similar age and gender who also shot off fireworks but didn't get injured.

In statistics, a theory that can be tested is called a hypothesis, or a theory you can prove wrong. For example, "witches cause global warming" can't be tested because you can't measure witchcraft. However, "global warming is associated with humans releasing CO_2 and methane" can be tested because you can measure levels of these gases.

Once you complete collecting your data, you make a hypothesis, such as "People who shoot off large fireworks are more likely to be injured than those who shoot off small fireworks." Another way to say this is: "There is an association between shooting off large fireworks and getting injured.

You can't test the hypothesis directly because statistics don't know about fireworks. But you can generate a null hypothesis, which says, "Any association is due to chance alone." Statistics can tell you how likely your associations are due to chance alone. A typical result is something like this. "There is one chance out of twenty that the size of fireworks and association is due to chance alone.

Don't worry if you are not clear on this. Most people live long and satisfying lives without understanding statistics. The important thing is to rely on people who do understand to tell you what is going on. In other words, Dr. Fauci of the National Institutes of Health provides better advice than Alex Jones or QAnon. When people say, "Do your own research," it doesn't mean visit a few conspiracy theory websites, it means read scientific publications and examine their statistics."

Our trainees came up with many hypotheses, mostly common-sense ideas based on the sentinel data and their general knowledge, including "bigger firecrackers lead to bigger injuries," "bigger injuries are associated with more tetanus," and "being drunk may lead to more injuries." My favorites are "eating sticky foods is associated with injuries" and "throwing lit firecrackers with your hand leads to injury."

Then the trainees fanned out to the major hospitals in Manila to find people with fireworks injuries and track them down to their homes and then talk to their neighbors and see if the neighbors used large fireworks, etc.

After a month, Conchy presented the results from the analysis to Manolet. Injured people were four and a half times more likely to have used big fireworks like super Lolo (grandfather) or baby dynamite.

Cases were five times more likely to have held lit fireworks in their hands and 3.6 six times more likely if they drank alcohol or were unsupervised children. Children weren't at higher risk if an adult supervised them. Older children and young adults were at higher risk if they were drunk or eating sticky food. Injured people were also more likely to have eaten sticky foods.

Budsy and I presented the results to Manolet. She said.

"The highest risk are unsupervised, drunken children eating sticky foods and throwing lit fireworks." She held out her hands, palms up in a "there you have it" expression.

Manolet ignored the joke. "I'll make you an appointment to see Dr. Bengzon. He'll want to know this."

Budsy and Conchy returned from the secretary's office shaken, as we all were when he talked to us, but the news was good. "He wants us to do a health education campaign before New Year's to bring down the injuries and tetanus. He gave us twenty thousand dollars."

Twenty thousand was more than chump change during those times, enough for serious TV time and newspaper space. We knew that we also could count on the health reporters to give us free coverage as well.

Budsy sent her nurses to set up surveillance sites in all the major hospitals in Manila, Cebu, and Mindanao. The nurses, trainees, and staff would be stationed in ERs. Budsy and I would drive around the city, checking on our sites. A haze was hanging over the city, so we asked the weather bureau, Pagasa, to gather air samples and measure particulates overnight. The name resembles *pag-asa*, Tagalog for "hope."

In November, we began our media blitz. During the first week of December, we conducted city-wide surveys and learned that nearly everybody had heard about our messages and that most could recite them. Everything was going according to plan.

We all spent New Year's Eve in ERs around the city. As the sun rose, we met at the Aristocrat, Manila's famous twenty-four-hour restaurant. The dining room took up a quarter of a city block. Exterior walls folded away so you could enjoy breezes from Manila Bay across the street.

Budsy wiped her brow with the back of her hand and said, "What a night! There seem to be more injuries than expected."

"Don't say that. Don't forget we ran a campaign to convince people not to blow off their hands."

She handed me the tall menu. The Aristocrat was like an enormous diner. You could get almost any Filipino dish there. I ordered my favorite, *calderetang kambing*, a Spanish stew with spicy goat meat and olives.

We agreed to buy breakfast for the trainees and nurses. As they trickled in, the story was the same: more and more injuries. We still had work to do. Dr. Bengzon expected a report on New Year's Day before noon.

A few of us headed for the office to put the data together and write the report. Each team entered its data on portable computers as soon as they completed the forms. Budsy and her nurses only had to combine the data in their big computer and generate tables and graphs.

I headed over to Pagasa to get the air pollution report.

A red-eyed weatherman showed us his equipment. It worked by blowing air through a filter. "Never seen anything like this," he said. About a half inch of soot was piled atop the filter. "The only thing I can tell you is the level was very high. Most big particles will be trapped in peoples' noses and throats. There must be plenty of little particles around five microns across."

In the Plague Branch, I learned that if you inhale particles bigger than five microns across, they will be caught in the upper airway. You get rid of them by blowing your nose or sneezing. Five-micron particles drift down into the lungs n to land in the tiniest tubes or bronchioles that lead to the alveoli, the tiny air sacs. This may cause severe coughs or asthma attacks. If the particles are plague bacilli, they will cause plague pneumonia, which is usually fatal. Particles smaller than five microns are so tiny that they usually drift in and out of the airways without landing anywhere.

The soot particles in the Manila air caused an increase in asthma and lots of coughs. I could testify to this, as I sometimes coughed up little globs of black mucus on New Year's Eve.

Back at the office, Budsy showed me charts of injuries. Everywhere, injuries soared as the night wore on. San Lazaro was the only place we had data from the year before. With many new hospitals, the total number of injuries went up sharply for every category—more fingers and hands blown off than before. Injuries per thousand people went down, but we were the only ones who seemed to notice. The raw numbers made better headlines, I guess.

Manolet and I called Dr. Bengzon at home and read him a press release based on the report. The secretary was not happy with the results of his twenty-thousand-dollar campaign. Worse, the media portrayed us as failures, not as people of goodwill trying our best, but as incompetent government bureaucrats.

A couple of weeks later, Mike Gomez popped into our office with a can of WD-40 and fixed the squeak in our door hinges. Mike was a funny guy and intelligent. He worked for Manolet in the Public Health Information and Education Service.

"Mike, do you have any idea why our health education campaign failed?"

He smiled tolerantly. "Your message was 'Don't blow off your fingers and hands, and so on.'"

"What's wrong with that?" I asked.

"Everybody already knew that. The problem isn't a lack of knowledge. It's that people don't apply that knowledge. You're scratching the wrong itch. You need to convince them they need to follow your advice."

I doubted it, yet he made sense. I replied, "People tell me we're trying to change basic Filipino culture."

Mike shook his head. "I hear that, too, but there's nothing un-Filipino about protecting your kids from blowing their fingers off. They're just blowing smoke to excuse themselves from doing nothing."

"So, Mike, what do we do?"

"Do what the tobacco companies do. Get an advertising agency."

Mike and I contacted several big agencies to see whether they'd create a campaign for us pro bono. The agency execs agreed to whip up some ads but pointed out that we'd still need to pay to put them on TV or in the papers. Mike went to work on the stations and newspapers, but only a few were willing to give us free space or time. Station managers and editors pointed out our campaign's failures from the year before, and they didn't want to waste time or space.

It was painful to hear, particularly because it was true.

The following New Year's, injuries fell 10 percent. Even better, the tetanus peak fell by nearly half. Still, both were unacceptable. Each year brought another slight decrease.

Then Budsy had an idea. "Filipinos love fireworks—the bigger, the better."

"Don't give me that cultural shit, Buds."

"Listen, Puti (my nickname, Puti, means white and usually is used sarcastically), open your mind for once. Fireworks are illegal, yet everybody from the police down ignores the law—including us. Every year, there's a race to sell bigger and better fireworks."

"OK." I looked at her carefully. "So what?"

"If we legalize fireworks, we can regulate them and make sure they don't make them bigger."

"Sounds crazy," I said, and yet it made an odd kind of sense.

Dr. Bengzon saw this right away. He went to bat for legalization and got it passed. The following year, injuries and tetanus dropped significantly, but significant peaks in injuries and tetanus still surfaced during the first week of January.

Fate took a hand. Dr. Bengzon decided to run for the

Senate. Polls showed he was the most popular cabinet member and that DOH had the most credibility of all government agencies. He looked like a shoo-in, but he wasn't. The Department of Agriculture sponsored a bill to double the pay of veterinarians. It passed, and vets then made almost twice the salaries of government doctors.

When DOH doctors appealed to Dr. Bengzon, he told them the government was short of money. "You'll have to wait until we refill the government's coffers."

He took a principled stand, but the doctors were furious, and many campaigned against him. In the end, he lost.

The new secretary was Dr. Juan Flavier, a colorful man with a Ph.D. from an American school of public health. He wasn't the bureaucrat or manager ARAB was, but he had other talents, particularly in public relations and motivating people. He brought in a woman named Suzy Pineda, who was a popular celebrity. Suzy once invited Budsy and me to appear on her radio show. When we stepped into the studio, she told me she would interview us both. I would have to speak Tagalog because most of her audience didn't speak English. I struggled but was clear enough that some listeners called in and asked me questions.

Dr. Flavier and Suzy negotiated with governors and mayors to put on huge fireworks displays in major cities. Admission was free, but police stood at the gates and prevented anyone from bringing in their own fireworks or alcohol.

Thousands of people from every big city attended the displays. Finally, the tetanus peaks disappeared. People still shot off fireworks, but few significant injuries occurred.

Looking back, we did change the culture, but it took a lot of people. We couldn't have done it without ideas and support from national politicians, mayors, and many others.

We didn't get it right the first, second, or third times, but we kept failing better and better, as they say. I think that's how all big ideas are made real.

My friends forced me to swallow a duck egg each New Year's Eve for seven consecutive years. I never developed a taste for them.

Some things can't be changed.

CHAPTER 15
ON THE VOLCANO

Mount Pinatubo was the site of the greatest volcanic eruption in the world in our lifetimes. On June 15, 1991, it exploded with the force of ten Mount Saint Helens, disgorging the most ash and gas since the storied eruption of Krakatoa in 1883. Pinatubo blew about twenty million tons of sulfuric acid into the stratosphere, lowering global temperatures by about two degrees centigrade for two years.

Don't get any ideas.

Fireworks were a minor problem compared with a volcanic eruption.

I first heard about Pinatubo when Dr. Bengzon called me to an urgent meeting.

An assistant met me at the entrance to his office and ushered me into a small windowless room where I would wait to be called into the secretary's office.

The room stank of tobacco smoke. I looked up to see a dark-skinned man wearing worn, stained fatigues sitting across the room. He wiped sweat from his forehead with the back of his hand. He smelled sweaty, too. A black, white, and red headscarf completed his appearance. He stared at me with hard black eyes.

He could only be a Moro rebel from the great forests of

Mindanao, the big southern island. Somebody had taken his weapons—a good thing, as Muslim rebels hated Christian Filipinos and Americans.

A small yellow light hung from the ceiling of the stuffy room. I felt a little ill from the smoke and reached over and turned on the fan. We didn't speak. He glared at me, and I watched him like a gazelle in a cage with a lion. I couldn't help but squirm as the clock ticked off the minutes.

Finally, an aide led me out and through the big mahogany doors of Secretary Bengzon's office. I stood beside his large mahogany desk. He didn't look up from the stack of papers he was reading and signing. I wondered whether there were any mahogany trees left in the country.

Eventually, he looked up, his face creased with a flicker of distaste. Beneath thick eyebrows, his eyes seemed to suck in all the light like black holes. He wore a handsome, formal *barong Tagalog*—a flowing white shirt with long sleeves. I looked down at my informal, lime-green barong. It was only slightly more formal than a T-shirt. He probably thought I was aping his culture.

"Dr. White, I'm in charge of negotiating with the rebels and bringing them back into society. I'm certain the American government is interested in this. Correct?"

I couldn't think of any reason the US government might care about this one way or another, so I stood silent, trying to meet his eyes and not look down.

"And I'm sure you know that I'm in charge of negotiating the removal of the American bases or a significant increase in the amount the Americans pay us for them. It will be in the Americans' interest to have inside information about my bargaining position.

"You're an American." It sounded like an accusation.

"Yes, sir."

"So, how do I know you're not a spy?"

"Sir, with all due respect, I can't prove I'm not a spy. If I were a spy, I'd deny it. Since I'm not a spy, I also deny it."

He had been sitting erect. If there's such a thing as sitting at attention, he was doing it. He smiled dryly. I think he was testing me.

He rose, led me to a chair by a coffee table, and sat across from me. "This is important. I want you to take careful notes."

I opened my notebook, hands slippery with sweat, and reached into my pocket for my pen. Jesus. It wasn't there. I couldn't ask him to lend me a pen, but he would notice if I didn't write anything.

"White." He paused. We both listened to the silence for a while. "Last week, the director of PhilVolcs, the seismological institute, called and gave me some news that involves you."

He glared.

"He told me there have been thousands of little earthquakes under Mount Pinatubo. He says that's a sign it will almost certainly erupt within the next six months. There might be tens of thousands of evacuees, and this department will ensure they are healthy. If they're not, we'll find ways to cure them. Manolet says you do a good job. I'm impressed when I see what your trainees have done to solve and stop epidemics. I've come to think of them as my crack troops."

"Thank you, sir." I scanned the coffee table and the carpet for a pen or pencil. Nada.

"Wherever the evacuees are sheltered, wherever they go, we need to protect them against disease. I'm told that in disasters in developing countries, more people die of infectious diseases than from the disasters themselves. This will not happen on my watch."

He looked at the blank page in front of me. "Are you writing any of this down?"

Exposed! He shouted, "Alma, get Dr. White a pen."

A pretty woman in her thirties stepped through the door

and handed me a pen. I scratched his orders down, carefully writing big so he could read them from across the table if he wanted to.

Dr. Bengzon said, "I'm impressed by the national surveillance system Budsy set up. I want her to use her nurses to set up a surveillance system for diseases among the evacuees and give me daily reports. I want you, Budsy, and your trainees to coordinate closely so we'll know their needs and can respond rapidly. You and the trainees will react promptly to stop any epidemics they find and keep them from spreading."

"Yes, sir."

"Good. Go see Mario, and he'll brief you."

I'd seen Mario Taguiwalo, the deputy secretary, many times since he hired me. Mario shared Dr. Bengzon's passion for improving the Filipino people's health, but his temperament couldn't be more different.

He smiled and leaned back in his chair. "Mark, I'm managing the whole government response, largely because of my work running the Baguio earthquake. Much of my success was due to you and your trainees' fine work."

"Thank you, sir. We'll do our best."

"Any thoughts on what will kill people after the eruption stops?"

"I looked up medical problems in disasters in developing countries. The biggest killers in the evacuation centers probably will be measles or diarrhea."

"Then we have a problem. The Aeta tribe lives way up the mountain. Over the years, the lowlanders—meaning us—took their land and drove them up the mountain, where it's pretty barren. They don't trust anybody, and I don't think they'll come down unless the volcano erupts. Then, assuming they don't die instantly, they'll come roaring down the mountain, and we'll have to take care of them. We'll stockpile measles vaccines at the Regional Health Office in Tarlac. Let me know what you need, and it'll be there. I'll make sure there are generators for the refrigerators to keep it from going bad if the power goes out."

I was impressed by Mario's clear vision and direct orders. "Yes, sir."

"Don't give me that shit. I'm Mario."

"OK, Mario."

We spent the following weeks reading about problems in evacuation centers and what to do about them. Budsy and I designed a surveillance system, and we worked with the people designing the centers to have a clinic in each center with one of Budsy's surveillance nurses. We stockpiled computers and paper, assigned nurses and doctors to each clinic, and waited. One night, we were in the office at 3:00 a.m. I went to Budsy's office and found she'd sent out for burgers and fries. They were limp now, the fries a greasy mess. It felt like there was sand around my eyeballs, but I went back to the office to work on the computer network for the surveillance system. I awakened on my couch, shoes still on, with rumpled clothes and stale breath. Budsy stood there, holding a cup of coffee. Her clothes and hair were perfect. I don't know how women do it.

We still weren't ready three weeks later, but it seemed we were getting things under control. Not the beginning of the end, but the end of the beginning, as Churchill said. We went home most nights now. I was up to six beers after dinner, and now I had to add Jack Daniels or vodka gimlets to get to sleep. The following day, Budsy and her deputy headed out to field-test the forms and data flow again. There was way too much data to share on the phone, and she expected that the phone lines would be down anyway, so somebody would need to drive to each evacuation center daily.

We still weren't ready when Mario called my office. "Mark, Rey Punongbayan, head of the Philippines Institute of Volcanology and Seismology, called five minutes ago with the news. The tremors under the mountain are getting bigger and closer together. There are now hundreds per hour. They say it's going to go off any minute."

Manolet told me Rey was the consummate volcanologist "who made volcanoes and earthquakes sexy." At this point, I found them sexy enough on their own.

We told the trainees and walked to the car. We'd sold our red sports car and bought a big silver Mitsubishi Pajero. Budsy had packed it weeks ago, like an expectant mother ready to go to the hospital. Pinatubo was three hours from Manila on the big four-lane divided highway. We were the only car going toward the mountain, and she floored it. I looked over her shoulder at the speedometer. It was touching a hundred. "God damn it, Buds, we aren't going to be any good to anyone if you kill us." She slowed down to ninety. I was grateful, but an endless traffic jam blocked the other side. It looked like a migration out of the Bible, with cars and jeepneys hauling luggage and packages tied to the tops. Farmers walked along the side of the road, driving their water buffaloes and cows.

I began to wonder whether we were going in the right direction.

Budsy looked out the window. "This is the real Philippines, green fields to the horizon, mango trees, and coconut palms. The blue skies."

The skies weren't blue for long. A typhoon blew up a few minutes before we reached Tarlac, the town at the foot of the mountain. It started to rain, and sheets of droplets slammed against our car amid lots of thunder, which was constant when we reached the Provincial Health Office (PHO). Sometimes a tremor occurred, and Budsy had to turn the wheel to keep us from veering off the road.

The rain on the windshield began to change from clear to black. Only later did we learn that the eruption was now spewing out the dark, gritty sand—volcanic ash.

Finally, Budsy swerved into the PHO parking lot, pumped the brakes, and slid into a parking spot right by the front door. She was a great driver. We pushed through the double doors. Conky Quizon, one of our best graduates, was in charge of the largest evacuation center. It would hold about ten thousand people.

She'd worked more than full-time for weeks, even though she was now very pregnant. Conky's door was open. Budsy entered first, then Conky stood, arching backward over her desk, feet spread wide. She said, "Ooh."

Conky's blouse hung open. Her belly pushed her skirt down. A stream of fluid trickled down her leg and onto the floor.

Budsy said, "You broke your water. We best get you to the hospital, or Mark and I will have to deliver you right here."

Conky grimaced and made a little laughing sound. "All we have to do is walk down the hall. If you'll support me." Budsy was, of course, already behind her. I stiffly walked up and reached a hand into her armpit on the other side. We staggered down the hall.

Conky puffed a couple of times. She said, "Don't forget you promised to fill in for me. You'll be in charge of the health of all the evacuees in Tarlac. Go see Tony. He's waiting for you."

As we pushed through the double doors and into the maternity ward, I said, "If it's a girl, you should name her Pinatuba."

Conky groaned. A nurse rushed up with a gurney. Conky lurched away from me. The nurse and Budsy helped her up.

Budsy returned and said, "Come on, genius, let's see Tony."

Walking down the hall, we peered out at the darkness every time we passed a window. The typhoon blew fine gravel, branches, and leaves against the rattling glass.

At the time, we weren't sure whether the volcano had started erupting. It had, of course.

Tony Lopez was, for my money, the best provincial health officer in the country. A tall, thin, thoughtful man, he waved us into the visitor's chairs opposite his desk. He slid some papers aside, walked around, sat on the front of his desk, and looked down at us.

He looked the worse for wear, with tired eyes and stooped shoulders. Finally, he spoke. "It's the Aetas; they're going to take the brunt of this."

Tony took out a handkerchief and wiped his brow. His phone rang, but he ignored it. "The Aetas are suspicious, so most of them ignored our warnings. We put the few who agreed to come down in Camp O'Donnell near the base"

I said, "Isn't Camp O'Donnell where the Japanese put the concentration camp after the Bataan Death March?"

"Yes. There's plenty of housing and services for large numbers of people. Good for concentration camps and evacuation camps."

"That's pitiful," Budsy said.

Tony smiled thinly, "Don't worry about history. Last week PhilVolcs enlarged the danger zone, so we moved the Aetas down to Camp Aquino, more than ten kilometers from the caldera. It's probably pretty safe for now."

He picked up a Styrofoam cup of cold coffee from the desk. Two more cups of indeterminate age sat near it. I felt depressed. Budsy stared skeptically at him. She said, "If they stay on the mountain, they'll burn up. What will happen to them when they come down?"

"In the short term, there will be plenty of room, food, and shelter in Camp Aquino. The governor is asking Manila for money to build houses and train them for jobs. That'll take a while."

Budsy said, "But Congress hasn't agreed."

"Not yet, but we think they will. What choice do they have?"

He slid off his desktop, bowed his head, and wiped his eyes with his hands. "I'll take you to my house and show you where the shower is. We start up the mountain after you clean up and change your clothes."

Budsy put out her hand with the palm out. "Stop right there. The mountain is erupting. Why would any sane person want to go up there?"

Tony had been putting papers into his attaché case. "Things are under control down here. I've sent medical teams high up in the mountains near the Aeta camps. They'll take care of any acute injuries, but they may need to come down fast. We'll be near O'Donnell, staying at my summer cottage. It's not far from here."

"Well, shit," Budsy said, "if you're going to throw us into the mouth of the volcano, there's no sense in changing our clothes. I can testify that Mark and I are not virgins, just in case you're getting ideas."

Tony smiled wearily, snapped his case shut, and led us out so we could follow his car.

We both knew we would have to go. It was unthinkable to refuse to take the risks others in the DOH were taking. A gaping hole of fear opened in my stomach. We'd spent months reading about volcanos and had a fair idea of what might be waiting up there in the rumbling and smoke.

The earth beneath the PHO was now trembling almost constantly, and black rain slanted against the windows.

We waited for Tony to take us to his home.

CHAPTER 16
IN THE HOT ZONE

We didn't wait long.

I sat in Dr. Lopez's office, picturing the earth below us. I imagined gigantic continental plates shoulder over each other as the magma squirted ever faster up toward us as the hole beneath Mount Pinatubo grew.

My reverie was interrupted by a knock on the door. A middle-aged man with a wrinkly face walked in. Tony said, "Budsy and Mark, meet Juan, my driver." Juan held out his hand to shake. It felt greasy and gritty. That was how the ash felt.

Budsy took a deep breath and led us out into the storm.

Tony's car was parked next to ours. They started first, and Budsy followed them up the narrow road clinging to the mountainside. The thundering was worse now. Still, we could see well enough to relax a bit. I tried to rest, but images of pyroclastic flows and surges painted themselves in my mind. They are the most dreaded effect of volcanic eruptions—rivers of superheated gas made of sulfur dioxide and rock roaring down mountainsides like freight trains at three hundred miles per hour. No way to run, no place to hide. That's what got the people of Pompeii. They didn't know what hit them, and neither would we. We'd be vaporized, but the rock would solidify around each of us, leaving a perfect mold. Perfect for archaeologists to make plaster statues of us. Cold comfort.

A loud chuff made us jump. The ash fall increased and blackened the air. We could barely see. A great tremor shook us sideways, near the chasm on the outside of the road. Budsy corrected, then nearly rear-ended Tony's car. We'd arrived.

Juan jumped out and led us with his flashlight to a parking space.

Tony was lighting kerosine lanterns inside the cabin as we quickly scampered in. Juan followed with the ice chest and a six-pack of beer. We had all the essentials for survival.

We stood with our feet apart to stabilize ourselves and shouted into each other's ears over the roaring.

"Tony," I yelled above the thundering, "How far up is the Aeta clinic?"

"A long way," he said vaguely.

"Hey, Tony." Budsy had the calm, patient expression you use when humoring a crazy person. "You think we might get a little pyroclastic flow?"

"Of course not. It'll be channeled into the valleys on either side of us. Ditto for lahar (rivers of boiling mud)."

Budsy eyed him. "So you thought this through before we left?"

"I checked the PhilVolcs maps. I wouldn't have brought you up if there was any risk."

Budsy looked up into his eyes. Deadly serious. "Tony, if it's not safe, we should go back now."

Juan opened the beers and handed them around. Every driver I knew drank a lot of beer when it was free. I held my bottle tightly and did some arithmetic. Budsy wouldn't drink any, so three were gone. That left nine, only two more for each of us. Shit. No help for it now. I'd have to economize. Or maybe I should drink as fast as possible and finish them before Tony and Juan drank it all.

We heard a noise outside. Could this be it? Budsy said, "Dios mío." She grabbed me in a tight protective embrace. She was a good woman, a great wife. I put down my beer, and we hugged close.

Budsy relaxed her embrace and sat back down with a thump when the cabin shook.

I didn't see my beer vibrating toward the edge of the table until Budsy yelled, "Hey," and snatched it from the very edge. Then the floor bumped up, and the roar increased to a deep scream from the earth's center. Finally, it quieted to a steady, thunderous grumbling.

It was impossible to make small talk, so we shouted back and forth about Tony's plans for evacuating the Aetas when the eruption chased them down. One of the many differences between the Aetas and me is that I was already scared enough to run down right then, but backing out was no longer an option. Even if I could persuade my brave companions to abandon our posts, the clouds of ash combined with the driving rain made it impossible to get anywhere, even on foot. Tony and Budsy went outside to check on the cars. They were gone a few seconds and returned, coated with ash.

"There's a big wind out there. The ash and rain are so thick, you can't see your feet, even with the flashlight," Tony said. "The Aetas will have to take care of themselves."

The door shook with a loud banging. A person coated with a crumbling layer of ash stood there. He swept ash out of his eyes and off his clothes. "I run the clinic near the Aeta village. It's bad up there," he said. "Red-hot rocks are falling and burning through the tents and hitting people. They're light—pumice, I think.

"I tried to get them to come down, but they're afraid. God help them."

The door opened again, and a skinny Aeta burst in. He was covered with gray ash and held the left side of his head with his hand. When the doctor pulled it off, we saw a deep purple bruise surrounded by a ring of angry red burn. "That's what the injuries look like," he said. He spoke the Aeta language and told the gray man the bandages were all used up. The man shook his head to show he understood. Then he was out the door. We looked after him and saw him running down the road, disappearing around a curve. I never saw him again. I hope he made it.

I pushed my chair back against the wall but didn't feel much more stable. I tried to get a hold of my nerves in this trembling, roaring world. Suddenly, a sharp pain split the left side of my skull in half as if someone had hit it with an ax. I've never had migraines, and if this is what they feel like, sufferers have my sympathy. An electrical buzzing reached out of the pain and made it hard to think—it seemed that part of my brain wasn't working right anymore. As a doctor, I prescribed two more medicinal beers, then added a third to be safe. Tony and Juan would have to take care of themselves.

As Budsy acidly predicted, the beer didn't help.

Or maybe it did. Even with the roaring and stabbing headache, I was suddenly very sleepy. I gave in to despair and fatalism as Budsy led me to the bedroom. We crawled under the blanket and wrapped ourselves in each other's arms.

I felt her lips against my ear. "If we have to die, let's do it together."

She pressed against me, and I felt her shaking. So was I.

I whispered, "Not yet, Budsy, not yet."

And we fell asleep.

CHAPTER 17
MORNING IN THE ASHES

Budsy kissed me awake. She wore a T-shirt and panties. Lovely.

She crept from under the blanket, slipped into her jeans, and ventured into the living room. It was profoundly quiet, broken only by the snowflake-like whisper of ash dropping in the misty rain. We weren't dead, but there was no light: ash covered the windows.

I lay trembling in the blackness. It felt like my heart had fallen down an elevator shaft. No matter how chaotic epidemics seem, I had the tools to find patterns that allowed us to stop them quickly. In the uncaring geological eruption, we were as insignificant as bugs on a windshield.

Buds returned in a few minutes with a cup of hot coffee. I didn't care that it was instant.

I went to the main room. My headache was gone, which was lucky because Tony and the doctor from the aid station were ripping up sheets for bandages. The sound would have sent me to the rafters if I'd had a migraine.

Budsy made scrambled eggs with garlic fried rice with fried fish. My favorite breakfast. The smell filled the cabin as we all wolfed it down.

Some Aetas knocked on the door, and Tony pointed the

healthy ones down the road. He brought in the injured. Most only had bruises that we could bandage. We needed to splint a few broken limbs, and several had coughing fits and shortness of breath. We helped Tony get the worst few into his truck. He told the doctor he'd be back. "Hang in a few more minutes, an hour max."

The doctor stared back in weary pain. "Fine," he mumbled. "Bring some doughnuts and real coffee." Napoleon said an army travels on its stomach. Public health runs on coffee and beer.

After an hour, enough people with severe injuries arrived for us to load up our SUV. Colorless morning light filtered through a flurry of ash drifting down. Budsy gingerly pulled into the stream of Aetas marching down toward safety.

I said, "Try not to bump so much. We have people with broken bones in the back seats."

"Screw you. The road disappeared under God knows how many feet of wet ash. It's a wonder I don't slide off the side and over the cliff."

She slammed on the brakes. Two men had jumped onto the hood to ride down. "Get out there and chase them off," she said.

I did. After that, she honked the horn whenever people got on the hood. She let two people ride outside on the running boards.

After slipping on and off the road for a terrifying eternity, we reached the big evacuation center at the large Philippine army base. It was in the middle of the parade grounds. Rows and rows of tents were set up, but as more people flowed in, it was clear that these tents could not accommodate them all, so the new families squatted in the rain. Health workers and soldiers brought out tarps. Beneath them, people huddled, shivering in the black rain.

Later that day, the rain stopped. Dr. Lopez and Conky had planned well. The health workers organized the evacuees and set up clinics and feeding stations. The army didn't want us to dig latrines, but the need was obvious now. We handed out shovels and showed some evacuees where to dig long trenches.

We drove on and dropped our load of injured Aetas off at the hospital, then looked around the wards for Conky. She must have delivered in the night. Except for the injured people we dropped off, the beds were empty. Finally, we found her.

She lay like a Madonna with her baby, Oyo, in her arms. She said, "As the deputy provincial health officer, I felt my duty was to stay here to avoid panic. It didn't work. Aside from us, there's only one other patient, and he's in a coma. His family is in Manila."

She looked at Budsy. "Will you be Oyo's godparents?"

"Of course."

After a few minutes, I asked, "When are you heading home?"

"Tomorrow. You look like you've been through hell," she said accurately. "Go to my house and wash off and get some rest." What a woman.

We found her husband sweeping a half inch or so of ash out the front door. He led us to a bedroom, then returned to sweeping. I had a couple of beers, and we slept again.

Back at Camp O'Donnell, the nurses and midwives prepared to immunize the evacuees for measles. Isolated populations like the Aetas don't get exposed to measles very often, so nobody is immune. They were all at risk, particularly those with malnutrition. Half of them could die, adults and children.

There was just enough time for the measles vaccine to keep people from getting sick, but we needed to start immunizing at once. We stood high in a reviewing stand with a commanding view. Budsy's nurses organized a line of midwives who marched through the crowd to vaccinate everybody. The jagged line moved slowly across and through the crowd. They were saving a lot of lives that day. Budsy and I looked at each other, hearts bursting with pride.

Then we ate lunch.

It was sardines. Sardines are the food the Philippine government stocks for disasters. I never liked them before, but now I find them delicious—probably the association with finally getting fed after long days working in the rubble of earthquakes and volcanic eruptions. However, the Aetas, living high in the mountains, had little access to fish and none to sardines. They didn't consider sardines food and often traded them for cigarettes. A brief fad spread, in which men used sardines for hair oil and decorations, but it didn't last. It was easy for them to subsist on canned meat, fruits, and vegetables. The US military donated thousands of MREs—trays of Meals Ready to Eat. I thought they tasted pretty good, and it was a nice change from sardines.

Budsy asked a nurse how the evacuees liked the MREs. "They eat some of the food. The men like the packets of matches."

"They're not eating them?" I asked, alarmed.

"No, they trade some of the MREs for cigarettes from the workers handing out the food."

At the end of the day, we joined the nursing supervisors to see that they had immunized hundreds of people. "Good job," Budsy said.

"The Aetas were afraid to take the shots or give them to their kids. Only the lowlanders accepted the injections, and many were vaccinated as children."

I drove to Manila the next day to give Dr. Bengzon the bad news and ask for help.

The secretary wanted to hear my report immediately. I parked next to a sports car with bullet holes in the side and a blood-soaked driver's seat.

I asked Manolet about the wreck. He said, "I asked Big Boy, the secretary's bodyguard. He said, 'Last night, they were coming back from a meeting with the NPA rebels and got stopped at an army checkpoint. Some jumpy soldiers shot first and didn't ask questions later.' They're going to tow it this morning.

"Time to go. The secretary is waiting for you."

Everyone in the outer office stared and moved out of the way as an assistant led me through the great doors to Dr. Bengzon's desk. He stood and, for the first time, smiled at me. He walked around to shake my hand and led me to the plush chairs by the coffee table.

"Alma, two coffees, and some *pandesal*." I loved the tasty, sweet-ish bread served for breakfast.

"And get Dr. White a pen and paper." He remembered. "I've got another appointment in twenty minutes, so tell me what's going on."

I told him about the devastation and the thousands of evacuees in Fort Aquino. "Sir, almost no Aetas took the measles vaccine. Measles is their greatest danger, and as many as half the cases might die."

He leaned back. "That's bad news. What do you recommend?"

I was ready, really ready, for this one. "Our only choice is to force the Aetas to take the vaccine. There's still time to stop the epidemic."

He stood up straight and glared down at me. My skin reddened, and I felt like I had a hundred-and-four-degree fever. Sweat trickled from my armpits and down my sides.

"White, don't they teach you ethics at CDC? Or in elementary school? You Americans!" he spat. The greatest curse in his vocabulary was to call somebody an American. "This disadvantaged minority, the original owners of these islands, to whom we owe an enormous debt, have the right to control their own bodies and their children. You Americans killed the

Native Americans and the slaves. I will not allow you to force anybody in this country to take medicine or anything else."

"Sir, what can we do to prevent hundreds of deaths? Surely we have an ethical duty to keep them alive."

"Of course. You must persuade them." He rose, and I followed unsteadily.

"I'm taking a lot of political heat from the fascists in Congress. They claim there are epidemics all over the place and want us to give them money to spend in their districts, and, of course, they will steal it or piss it away to their friends."

A week before the eruption, a restaurant donated some contaminated meals. I said, "Sir, we only found a single epidemic in an evacuation center in Manila. Our trainees closed the restaurant until they cleaned up their act."

"I know. I appreciate your trainees' fine work." No mention of my fine work, but I could hardly expect that now —or maybe ever.

He stood up. "I need daily reports. For each evacuation center, I want to see the rates of diseases every week. Give me tables and graphs for each disease, and I want to see the numbers of cases on each week's graph."

"But, sir, there are nearly sixty sites. It'll take forever to make all those graphs."

He reached past me and swung the door open. "We pay you an arm and a leg, more than I get as a cabinet secretary. I don't care if you have to stay up all night. Find a way."

He shouted for an assistant, and one instantly appeared, took my arm, and led me away. I heard Dr. Bengzon slam the carved mahogany doors behind me.

CHAPTER 18
BLOWGUN LESSONS

I n the first weeks after the eruption, we had good news for Dr. Bengzon. The amazing thing was that only a few people died in the immediate aftermath, mostly from the weight of wet ash collapsing roofs on them. The ash was several feet thick and heavy with rainwater. Many slipped and fell to the ground while cleaning ash off roofs fell from were injured. Most of the people at risk voluntarily evacuated to safety, and Aetas ran down during the eruption and avoided the worst damage. This was a triumph for the Philippine government's warnings and preparations.

Two days after Conky delivered Oyo, she took over supervising the evacuation centers. What a woman!

By then, the sandy, wet ash had stopped falling, but several feet covered everything.

As far as I could see, no lava was flowing from Mount Pinatubo, but thick, boiling lahar oozed down the slopes and into rivers, overflowing the banks. Budsy and I were distressed when we saw a water buffalo caught in the lahar, screaming in pain. There was no way to get near it, and it suffered until somebody shot it.

One sunny morning, I took a walk over what had been the richest rice fields in the country. Now it was an endless lunar plain of cracked, dry ash and lahar from horizon to horizon. Lahar had oozed out of rivers and buried the land. The rice was in the darkness four or five feet below, smothered, crushed, and burned. In the distance, I saw another person wandering, probably thinking the same thoughts. I guess we both felt a need for company and walked toward each other for the next half hour across the vast wasteland. The trees were long gone, except for occasional tall stumps standing like broken ancient columns. Once in a while, I noticed the absolute stillness. No songs from birds, croaking frogs, or the whispering of leaves. Only the dusty wind rustling by.

My fellow searcher turned out to be an American from the US Department of Agriculture, advising the Philippine government on how to recover the land for crops. He had thick gray hair and was wearing a neatly buttoned but weathered shirt that had once been tan or white, and his hands were strong and calloused. For years, the sun had burned his profoundly wrinkled face deep red.

I said, "I suppose this will turn into good agricultural soil in a couple of years. I heard volcanic soil is really rich. Do you think the farmers will be able to increase their yields?"

He glared. "Don't you know anything about soil microbiology?" he spat.

I was annoyed. "I'm a doctor, an infectious disease specialist, and I know a lot about microbiology."

"Really?" His bright-blue eyes were no longer appraising but disgusted.

I had imagined we were the last two men in the world and would find common cause in a post-nuclear wasteland. Now I realized we would have killed each other. "Really," I said. He would have washed out of medical school after two days.

He sneered. "If they taught you anything important, you'd know that soil is made of microorganisms—fungi, yeast, actinomycetes, bacteria, worms, and so on. The minerals are inert, mostly just the skeleton of the soil."

I did seem to remember something about this. "OK, but bacteria and fungi grow pretty fast. *E. coli* doubles every twenty minutes. How many months do you think it will take before they can plant rice again?"

"Decades. These people are screwed. I feel for them, but there's nothing anybody can do."

"Why not sow germs into the soil and speed things up?"

He turned and walked back toward the horizon where his trek had begun. I opened my mouth to say goodbye, but he didn't look back.

Back in Manila, it was easier to automate making surveillance tables and graphs for Dr. Bengzon. The nurses entered the data from the clinics and copied it onto diskettes. Drivers took the disks to my trainee Sonny Magboo and me every day. We sucked them into a report writing program and printed about fifty pages for the secretary. After a few days of brain-crushing programming, we got the system to run automatically.

And it worked for several weeks. Dr. Bengzon sent us a message complimenting us.

Also, one of our students, Rio Magpantay, came from the Region III Office, which included all the provinces directly affected by Pinatubo's eruption, and was familiar with the Aetas. Rio was one of our success stories. Not only did he become regional director, but he later ran a nightclub that had some terrific acts. Rio knew several Aetas and tried to convince them to accept vaccinations.

He said, "In Region III, we call the Aetas the *kulots*. It means curly, after their hair. They look more like the people in New Guinea than like us Malays."

After talking with several Aeta chiefs, Rio said, "Dr. White, I can't seem to get through to them." He also knew some anthropologists, none of whom could convince the Aetas.

None of us could think of how to prevent the disaster we saw coming.

Then another disaster struck. Sonny walked into my office and said, "Houston, we've got a problem."

"What?" I tried to speak in a slow, calm voice, like airplane pilots when announcing the engines had just shut down but telling the passengers not to worry.

Sonny brushed his thick black hair out of his earnest, dark-brown eyes. "It looks like a virus."

"Did you run the antivirus programs?"

"Of course. They didn't find any problems."

Terrible news. If we lost our whole data set for all the camps from these past weeks, we wouldn't be able to deliver the graphs Dr. Bengzon wanted. Failure was not an option.

It was already seven in the evening. Sonny and I ordered some burgers and went to work. Fortunately, we had the Norton Utilities program. It allowed us to do absolutely anything with disks and drives. We began looking at an infected diskette line by line, scanning screen after screen of hexadecimal numbers, like "8AE, BEF," etc. Occasionally, we would see words interspersed.

After a couple of hours and five or six cups of coffee, we found the line, "Bwa, ha, ha. Courtesy of the geniuses at Adamson University." Those snot-nosed college-student bastards.

Sonny and I checked a few more disks and found the virus in the same place. Fortunately, I knew how to write programs in the C language that Bell Labs used to control big computers. I wrote a little C program to delete the virus from the disks. By morning, we had cleaned the hard drives and diskettes.

Dr. Bengzon received his reports on time.

The camps near the mountain now contained approximately one hundred thousand evacuees. After a couple of weeks, the incubation period for measles, the epidemic started. Conky took me on a tour of the clinics. It was ghastly.

She introduced me to an Aeta child about ten years old. "They all look like this, pops," she said. I thought there might be a note of accusation in her voice. I tried to talk to him, but he didn't speak Tagalog, let alone English. I think he wanted to greet me, but he fell into a spasm of brassy, dry coughing. He was covered with red spots. When I looked in his mouth, his tonsils were huge and covered with pus. I feared he might be lapsing into pneumonia, a frequent complication that's often fatal.

Jesus. Couldn't I have done something to prevent this? Probably if I'd tried harder, pushed harder, and found more epidemiologists, anthropologists, or missionaries. Maybe we could have gotten troupes of actors to show the Aetas what would happen. I could've stood up on the stage and taken measles immunizations to show them they had nothing to fear. Epidemiologists did this with great success with smallpox in India. I should have thought of all these things and more.

But I hadn't.

In the end, 464 people, mostly Aetas, got measles, and 107 of these (23 percent) died. It was my fault. Instead of trying everything to save the Aetas, I was back in Manila with Sonny, writing computer programs and reports and rooting out computer viruses.

Sometimes I wake up on hot nights, sweating and trembling. I think I can see the faint outlines of the 107 dead Aetas drifting slowly around the room in the shadows. There's a Yiddish saying that a doctor isn't really good until he has filled a cemetery. By that standard, I'm a great doctor.

The following day, Dr. Bengzon summoned me to his office. Dread and numbness swirled through my mind.

Bengzon was a passionate and complex man. He studied in Jesuit schools and graduated from Ateneo de Manila, started by missionaries five hundred years before Harvard came on the scene. He nearly took religious orders but backed out just before the initiation ceremony. After medical school at the University of the Philippines, Dr. Bengzon studied in Germany, the US, and the prestigious Montreal Neurological Institute. A brilliant neurologist, he practiced at Medical City, the elite hospital. It nearly closed because it was losing money in the chaos of the failing Marcos regime. He took over the administration and turned it around in a single year. Dr. Bengzon was one of the best managers I've seen.

When Marcos declared martial law, Dr. Bengzon joined the political opposition and organized the Conveners' Group, which united opposition groups against the dictator. They chose Cory Aquino to run against Marcos. The rest is history.

I became part of Dr. Bengzon's history when Alma led me through his mahogany doors. He stood up, towering above me in his immaculate formal barong. I stood in front of his big desk and leaned against the edge to keep from shaking so obviously.

"Well?" he snarled.

I looked down, partly to avoid his blazing black eyes. "I'm sorry, sir. So sorry. We did everything we could, but they refused to let us vaccinate their kids." I knew enough not to remind him that he refused to allow me to force them to take the vaccine.

"Sorry? You're sorry? Over a hundred Filipinos under your care are dead, and you say you're sorry?"

"I failed, sir. I'm ashamed."

For the next ten minutes, he screamed and raged at me. I'm sure the people in the outer office were deafened.

"You know what you are, White? You're a murderer. A murderer, standing in my office."

I'll never forget those words. They hide in some dark closet in my memory and sometimes pop out like monsters.

He roared for what seemed like an eternity but was probably a couple of minutes.

He seemed to be running out of breath when his office door opened, and Alma looked at him. He snorted and sat down. She led me out. Bless that woman.

Guilt fastened itself like a vise to my abdomen and brain. I found my friend Manolet and choked out the story, wiping away the tears with the backs of my hands.

"This is great news." Manolet smiled. "He never talks to foreigners like that, only Filipinos. Don't you see? He's accepted you as one of us. I've never seen this before. It's a high honor."

"Even so . . . ," I began.

"If you want to immigrate, I know he'd support you."

I sniffled and left, dazed, bumping into his office door frame.

I threw myself into working at the camps with the Aetas. It was the least I could do. Near the end of my penance, I was working my way through the big crowd of Aetas when an old man approached me. Sun and rain had wrinkled his face like a raisin beneath curly black hair. He carried a long blowgun, the kind they used to shoot birds in the forests. He talked to the translator, who told me the old man wanted to sell it. I smiled gratefully and offered him several times what I thought it was worth. The wrinkled old guy probably had no idea about money.

He smiled, walked about fifteen feet away, and asked some kids to stand up a cardboard box target. The translator said, "He wants to show you how to use it."

He lifted the tube to his lips and opened his mouth to show me he was blocking the opening of the blowgun with his tongue. Then he put the feathered dart into the blowgun and blew. It made a *thwwt* sound, followed by the satisfying, solid *thunk* of the dart piercing the center of the target. I gave him the money and shook his hand. Trying to buy off my guilt, I guess. He grasped my wrists and pulled me close to his sweaty body. I held my breath.

I took the tube and a handful of feathered darts and backed away. The crowd surrounded us, and people pushed closer. They wouldn't let me through. The old man motioned me closer, took the blowgun, loaded it, then gave it to me.

Oh no, he wanted me to shoot it.

I looked at the hundreds of eager and amused faces and took the tube. If I missed the target, which seemed to be shrinking, I'd hit someone in the crowd. Jesus, I could kill another Aeta. Did the Aetas poison their darts?

The old Aeta coughed. He probably had TB. Maybe he had some nasty infection around his gums. In any case, I had no choice. I lifted it to my mouth with trembling arms, pasted my tongue over the wet opening, and blew. The tube wheezed, and the dart fell about three feet in front of us. The crowd exploded in applause and laughter. Several kids opened their mouths and showed me their tongues.

With the next try, the dart sailed past the target. The crowd threw themselves down and away, laughing. The Aetas had great reflexes.

I hit the target on my fifth try, and the crowd let me escape. I still have the blowgun in the attic, and every few years, I shoot it to keep up my skills.

No more epidemics broke out among the evacuees, and we gradually decreased the frequency of reports to once every other week. Still, Dr. Bengzon insisted we continue. Over the ensuing months, the government built concrete houses for the Aetas, who were getting fat on the sacks of rice and vegetables that arrived twice a week.

We finally convinced the secretary to let us stop the surveillance when we saw the Aetas putting up TV antennas. The ash didn't turn into fertile soil until a decade later, and it began to yield huge rice crops again. By then, the evacuation centers had turned into little communities of concrete houses.

The government had given the Aetas deeds to the homes and land to grow rice on.

Over the years, some Aetas moved back to the mountain forests, while others remained and farmed, and a few went to school. One even got a medical degree.

For centuries, the Aeta tribe had been dying out. The volcanic eruption killed some, but it improved the lives of many others.

CHAPTER 19
MY LIFE AS A SPY

When I started in CDC's Epidemic Intelligence Service, they cleared the auditorium and set up tables. Applicants to join walked from table to table as the line snaked around. It was like registering for courses in college. At one table, a guy in a suit asked me to sign a form. "It says you're not a spy working for a foreign power," he said.

"If I were a spy, I'd say no. If I say yes, it would prove I'm a spy. Does anybody ever check yes?" I asked, pen dangerously close to checking the yes box.

His face twisted in a look of annoyance and disgust. "Sign the fucking form."

I signed the fucking form.

The next time I was asked about spying was in the Philippines after I'd worked for the Department of Health for six months or so. I walked past Lhod, our secretary's desk. She looked up and asked me, "Kuya (brother) Mark, are you a spy?"

"Lhod, of course, I'm not a spy. No matter what I say, it looks like I'm guilty. It's like asking, 'When did you stop beating your wife?'"

She stared hard directly into my eyes. "Well, are you a spy?"

"No, I'm not."

"That's what I thought you'd say." She looked down, a curtain of long black hair covering her face. I looked around and saw two people looking in from the hall listening, their faces expressionless.

To paraphrase Dustin Hoffman in "Little Big Man," I thought that was the end of my spy period. Then the phone rang one morning as Budsy and I were getting dressed for work. I picked up and Lhod shouted into my ear, shrieking and crying. "I can see out my window. They're dropping bombs on Malacañang Palace. They're killing President Aquino! You've got to stop them."

"Jesus, Lhod, this is terrible."

"Call your friends at the embassy. Call the spies! Call anybody who can help!" Her voice rose to a keening cry. " They're killing her!" She hung up.

I looked at Budsy, who could hear Lhod screaming from across the room. I said, "Sounds like another coup attempt. She's either hung up or dropped the phone."

"Or the rebels cut the phone lines," she said and headed downstairs to turn on the television, leaving me alone in a humming, tense silence. I felt like somebody had punched me in the belly. I doubled over and felt tears trickling down my cheeks.

I wished I had a friend at the embassy, but there was little reason they should notice me. If they thought of me at all, it was as a scruffy hanger-on. I had a boss at USAID, the US Agency for International Development, but he thought I had "gone native," which I took as a compliment. Anyway, the ambassador would probably not call an epidemiologist for advice on what to do in a coup attempt.

The New People's Army was active during these unstable times. They didn't like the US Navy Research Unit (NAMRU), which was at the other end of the DOH compound from the FETP office. NAMRU had a long and distinguished history. They developed Oral Rehydration Fluid (ORS), which has saved hundreds of millions of cholera and diarrhea patients over the years. I don't think the NPA was aware of this. I called NAMRU one day and learned that Americans were all "working from home."

Eventually, I pried the truth out of them. A carload of Americans was exiting the compound when a garbage truck pulled up in front of them and dumped its load. Instantly, an old lady began picking through the trash. A big car pulled in behind them. The navy guys knew where they were, the kill zone. Sure enough, a motorcycle pulled up next to them, and the driver aimed a huge revolver through their window. The motorcyclist cocked the gun, gave them a smile and a thumbs-up, then roared off.

Later that afternoon, a politician was assassinated using the garbage truck tactic.

They were practicing on the navy guys.

After Lhod called, Budsy turned the TV to the ABS/CBN network. Their studio was only a few blocks from Malacañang. We saw the wide street Epifanio de Los Santos (EDSA). In the background, we saw the palace. The street was empty, blocked by two rows of huge concrete barricades with nervous soldiers of the Presidential Guard, rifles ready, peering out.

An announcer said they were replaying a video from earlier in the morning. A green army helicopter hovered over the palace, moving slightly as the pilot made corrections to keep the wind from blowing them away from their target. You could see dark objects falling toward the roof. Bombs. Then a little plane appeared and seemed to chase the helicopter away. While the air force had maintained its pusillanimous policy of neutrality, some heroic recruits must have flown their trainer from some distant base to protect the palace. Still, a trainer wasn't going to stop the ant-like column of soldiers pouring down the street like a flood of brown.

Budsy looked up from the TV red-eyed. "I'm too upset to go to work." So was I. We weren't afraid for ourselves. We were worried for Mrs. Aquino and the peaceful revolution she'd led—and that we'd crossed the Pacific to join.

We sat in the living room, growing depressed, drinking coffee and eating toast, the traditional food served at Filipino funerals.

An earthshaking explosion somewhere behind our house rattled the windows and sent glasses and cups skittering off the table. "Maybe it's some kind of earthquake," Budsy yelled. We'd better get outside." We ran through the front door and stood amazed as two American Air Force fighter jets swept past us, roaring and screaming just above the trees and houses. We ducked down with our hands over our ears. Of course, it didn't help. Under the wings were muscular missiles and fat ugly bombs. Two or three under each wing. These big bastards meant business. They roared off. Minutes later, they swooped barely above the heads of the rebel soldiers, then made a heart-stopping sharp loop and bore back down in what looked like a bombing or strafing run. The column broke into dozens of little lines disappearing down side streets. The siege on the palace was over. The jets pulled up and disappeared into the clouds.

The rebel officers apparently got their troops under control and led them away toward our subdivision. They passed an annex of the embassy. One sour soldier tossed a grenade over the fence. It landed in front of the medical clinic and blew up the doctor's car.

This genius act helps explain why all those coup attempts failed.

CHAPTER 20
THE FOUR HORSEMEN

T he last coup attempt was in 1989. Budsy and I were pinned down at home, assuaging our jitters by enjoying a breakfast of dried fish and *longganisa*, a sausage containing mystery meat, probably 80 percent fat, and God knows what else. It tastes great. I was chewing a bite when the phone rang, and I left the table to answer.

It was Susan, my case officer in Atlanta. "Did you read about the Ebola epidemic in Reston, Virginia?"

"The newspapers haven't made it through the roadblocks. All they show on TV is the coup. Sorry to hear about Reston. How many people are sick? You folks in Atlanta have work to do." The smell of coffee drifted from the kitchen.

Her reedy voice traveled across the Pacific into my ear. "It's only monkeys so far."

"So it's an epizootic." An epizootic is an epidemic among animals. I didn't need to know about monkeys in Virginia. Worse, Susan liked to talk, and she sometimes took a long time to get to the point. I shouted to Budsy to bring my coffee.

"Yes, and you have even more work than we do."

My chest tightened. "What do you mean?"

She dropped her voice. "The monkeys come from the

Philippines, from an export facility about an hour and a half from Manila."

Fuck. Fuck. Fuck.

Budsy arrived with the coffee. "Bring the whole pot and some aspirin."

She snuggled down next to me to listen.

There was rasping breathing on the phone. Susan said, "Are you still there? Any unusual sickness there?"

I swallowed and said, "No, but anything could be happening out there. We won't know it until after the coup."

She digested this for a few long seconds. "Now, I'm going to transfer you to the Special Pathogens Branch. I think you'll want to talk to them."

"Thank you. I'll be waiting right here." Her phone clicked as she put me on hold, leaving me to listen to the faint hiss of the lines across the Pacific Ocean.

Budsy poked my arm. She dug elegantly manicured nails into my skin. "Ebola here? Don't half the patients bleed to death?"

"Yep. It's horrible. Raging fevers, liver failure, kidney failure, bleeding into the stomach, bowel, skin, brain, lungs." I knew a lot about Ebola. I'd always dreamed I could cap my career with an Ebola epidemic. Now it seemed like a nightmare.

She asked, "Do you think it'll make it to Manila?"

"How many people live here?"

"About nine million." She blinked, then set her mouth.

My stomach clenched painfully. I felt a burning in my chest. The coffee must be washing back up—or I had a heart attack. At least I wouldn't have to deal with Ebola. Unworthy thought. I felt my face redden.

Budsy placed a warm hand on my arm. It felt good. "One good thing about being a Catholic is you learn a lot of scripture."

"You're not going to try to get me to pray, are you?"

"No. Do you remember the Four Horsemen of the Apocalypse?"

The phone clicked and went dead. Our exchange was in Makati, in rebel territory. CDC would call us back if the rebels hadn't cut the lines.

"Refresh my memory."

"Plague rides a pale horse. The others are famine, war, and conquest."

"Thanks for sharing."

Budsy said, "Remember the Spanish flu? It killed millions of people."

"We don't have time for more history. I need to call Manolet."

She looked serious. "The Spanish flu was spread when soldiers carried it around the world. Now, we have two of the four horsemen, plague, and war. What if Ebola infects the rebels, and they spread it to Manila?"

The phone rang. It felt like an axe splitting my head.

"Mark White," I answered, hoping to show a good, can-do attitude.

"John Snow here. Special Viral Pathogens." His voice sounded like Richard Burton's, deep, sonorous, and in control.

"Boy, am I glad to hear from you. We need you to help investigate ASAP. As soon as we finish the call, I'll call the Secretary of Health and get him to invite you." This was important. CDC teams can't go anywhere without an invitation from the local government. It goes double for foreign countries.

"Well, there're a couple of things we have to get out of the way first."

He sounded like a bureaucrat when I needed Seal Team Seven. My guts tingled with irritation.

"What do we have to get out of the way? Here's the situation. I've got myself, my boss, my wife, and twenty trainees to stop this epidemic before it gets to Manila. It's probably heading this way now. If you leave today, you can be here in twenty-four hours, thirty-six, tops."

"I understand your concern," he said distractedly. "The first problem is that I don't have a budget for this. You'll have to pay for our team out of your budget."

I partially suppressed a scream. "I run a training program. Our budget is peanuts. Bupkis. There's no way we could pay for your team."

"Well, I'll see what I can do."

I winced. I wasn't asking now. "Do that. You said there were two problems."

"The second is there are no flights to the Philippines. All airlines are grounded until the coup is over."

Anxiety turned into depressed acceptance. "There's no way you could at least send us some of those space suits you wear when you work with Ebola?"

"No chance. You don't need them anyway. I've done outbreaks in Africa with paper gowns and masks. No problem."

No problem? Even in my numb state, I felt sweat running down my forehead and armpits. "Can you at least send me a questionnaire so I can use the same methods you guys do?"

"We don't have standard questions." This guy was worthless. No help at all.

He continued. "Each outbreak is different, so you have to design the study and control measures to fit the situation on the ground."

"Fine. That makes sense. Can we talk about this now?" Budsy slipped a legal pad and pencil into my hand. She was so competent.

"Sorry, I've got a meeting. Email me your design and questions, and you'll have my comments and corrections in the morning."

"We're twelve hours different from you. It's already tomorrow morning here. We have to start right now."

"OK, I'll stay up and send the comments. Can you try to make it quick? It's my wife's book group night, and I have to get the baby to bed. Hurry up."

"OK. Just in case something comes up, like a thousand cases, can I have your home number?"

"Tomorrow morning."

"That's tonight here."

"Whatever. Goodbye."

We called Manolet, and it took us only an hour to design the survey. I emailed it to Snow in Atlanta. A half-hour later, he sent back comments. Most were minor.

For the first time that day, I felt relief. Things just might be coming under control.

When we called Manolet to tell him CDC approved our questionnaire, he said, "What a nightmare. I called Dr. Bengzon. I doubt he'll let us bring in American experts unless things are desperate. You know how much he hates Americans."

I said, "Yes, I know.

"Budsy and I will get our best trainees and head out first thing in the morning. I think you should stay with the department and the other trainees in Manila. You know, in case we get sick."

"OK, that sounds like a plan," he said. I listened hard for a tone of relief in his voice, but he was all business.

Budsy stood, thinking. She said, "Conchy's our best. She did a great job in Baguio. We probably ought to bring Betsy, too. She's a vet, and she handles herself well. You call. I'll get hold of the office staff and arrange a vehicle and supplies."

"Got it," I said.

Conchy picked up the phone on the second ring. I told her what was going on.

She said, "What time shall I be in the office?"

I'd expected no less. Conchy was a tough cookie and no stranger to danger. In Marcos's time, she was in the opposition, hunted by Marcos' soldiers in the northern mountains.

Next, we called Betsy. Before joining us in the FETP, she trained as a veterinarian and worked at the Research Institute for Tropical Medicine, the Filipino equivalent of the US NIH.

When Betsy picked up the phone, I explained the situation. She laughed. "Dr. White, nobody got us in messes like this before you came. Of course, I'll come."

"Fine. Your house is on our way, so we'll pick you up at about eight."

"Be careful of rebel roadblocks."

"We will."

In the evening, she called back. "You know I have a newborn baby, right? Will this be safe for her? Of course, I'll leave him with the *yaya* (nurse)."

I'm ashamed to say I reflexively answered, "Of course, you and the baby will be fine."

I should've called her back to tell her there was a risk, but I stifled my conscience under a few beers and tried to sleep. Even so, the occasional gunshots from the coup in Makati and explosions kept us awake. I might have slept through it if Buds hadn't hidden the last beer.

In the morning, Budsy and I put on jeans, T-shirts, and running shoes.

We would be ready for fight or flight. If it came to meeting Saint Peter, I was sure he'd understand.

The truck arrived right on time. Everybody trooped out for coffee and a last-minute rest stop. Budsy checked we had enough masks and gowns, needles and syringes, blood tubes and collection bottles, and an ice chest labeled with the international symbol for biohazards, which shows a circle with three menacing fountains shooting out.

Unfortunately, the fighting was directly between us and

the monkey export facility. Vic, our driver, said, "Don't worry, I'll take a shortcut around the rebels."

I said, "Thanks, Vic." He was a nice guy.

About two miles from our house, Vic steered us directly toward the Makati office towers, where you could see rebel soldiers looking down from roofs or leaning out of windows, following us with their guns. Some waved. They only allowed ambulances and food delivery trucks in and out of the city.

They seemed right at home. The night before, they'd treated themselves to five roast suckling pigs.

CHAPTER 21
MONKEY BUSINESS

Betsy looked back as the towers of Makati disappeared behind us. "Thank God that's over with."

Conchy's mouth turned into a little smile. "Yes, what a relief we only have to deal with an Ebola epidemic." She relaxed and put her head back against the seat. Conchy's the kind of fearless person you want on your team.

I watched a tire roll past us on the highway. I said, "Some poor bastard lost his tire."

Vic laughed, then held the wheel tightly as our truck sloughed off the side of the road. He managed to get us stopped before we hit the deep ditch.

"What's so fucking funny?" Budsy snarled. "You could have killed us. Don't you ever do maintenance?"

Vic opened his door. "Dr. White, can you help me get the tire?"

We jogged up the road to rescue our escaped wheel. As we rolled the tire back to the car, he said, "They make me take the car to the motor pool for service. Those bastards steal as much as they can, even nuts and bolts. I'm sure they got the lug nuts."

Between us, we got the truck up on the jack and scavenged some nuts from the other wheels. Budsy glared at our handiwork. "Great, now all four wheels will fall off."

Vic cringed. "I'll drive slow until we get to a gas station where we can get more nuts."

A half-hour later, we were at the gates of the export facility. A man in a T-shirt and jeans welcomed us. It was a T-shirt-and-jeans place.

"I'm Jose Mercator. This is my place." He smiled. "You must be Betsy." I realized we were now on Betsy's turf. As the vet, she contacted him and arranged for our visit.

Betsy smiled and shook his hand. "Any unusual deaths?"

Jose glanced at the ground. "We lose about 10 percent while fattening them up for shipping."

Betsy said, "Must be traumatic, getting trapped and shipped to Manila."

Betsy had made us an important friend.

He watched as we took out our gowns, masks, and paper shoe coverings.

Conchy said, "What about the staff? Anybody sick or not showing up for work?"

"Nope."

"We'd like to fill out a questionnaire on everybody who works here, including you."

Jose smiled. "Of course. Let me show you around."

The moment we walked in the door, a chorus of hooting and jabbering exploded from the cages. The monkeys looked to be about four feet tall. I later looked them up on Wikipedia. It said they were about two feet tall. Ours looked taller. They had long tails and short, muscular arms and legs.

Jose said, "You can tell the males because they have side whiskers."

Budsy said, "You can tell the males because they all have erections."

"That, too," he said. "They don't normally see women."

"These bastards are strong. And watch out for those teeth. Remember, they crush crabs for a living."

He was not exaggerating. The monkeys had huge yellow fangs dripping with saliva.

Budsy stared at the monkeys. "The teeth might not be the worst. There might be Ebola virus in the saliva."

Jose smiled indulgently. "We hardly ever get bitten, but it sometimes happens when one escapes."

Conchy said, "Do they ever get out of the building?"

"Of course, but we catch them."

"How?"

"We put a banana in a bottle and tie it to a post. The monks reach in and can't get the banana out. Monkeys are so greedy that they won't let go. We just grab them."

Betsy stepped forward. "We'll need a table to hold them while we take blood."

"I'll get a couple of guys to help you."

Conchy said, "Before we start with the monkeys, we'd like to take blood on everybody who works here.

Jose held his arm out, then shouted, "Everybody come here. These doctors need to ask you some questions." He smiled. "No sense in telling them about the blood samples until they're already here."

The men all denied illness. Clearly, they liked working here. At least a quarter were missing the last joint of one or two fingers.

Betsy said, "Let's start with the sick monkeys."

Two men disappeared and returned carrying a big cage. Budsy laid blue plastic sheets over the table. The guys reached into the cage and wrestled the monkey out. They pinned it flat on the table.

Budsy handed Betsy a syringe and an alcohol wipe. "I've bled dogs, cats, water buffalos, and pigs. But never a monkey."

"How hard can it be?" I asked.

Betsy looked at me with eyes that were wells of contempt.

She stepped forward, washed the skin on one side of the monkey's neck, and plunged in a needle. When she pulled back on the plunger to suck out blood, it was dry. She'd missed. The femoral veins in the groin are usually easy, but she missed them, too.

The monkey snarled and screeched more each time she stuck it. The handlers' eyes seemed to bug out more as the animal strained against them.

Everybody looked at me. I shrugged. "How about a fresh syringe and needle for good luck?"

Budsy had one ready.

First, I tried all the deep veins, as Betsy had. Nothing. The monkey snorted and seemed to be foaming at the mouth. I didn't want to kill the poor, vicious thing.

In the end, I went to the old familiar cephalic vein in the arm you use in people. I filled a tube on the first try.

I'm sure the monkey was relieved that the torture session was over. The handlers opened the cage door, and it rushed in.

I put my arm up and wiped the sweat from my forehead. Budsy reached up and pulled it away. No sense in risking getting an Ebola infection.

Betsy tried the next monkey and quickly got blood, so she took over bleeding the monkeys. In an hour, we were back on the road. Vic had bought lug nuts by then. This time he gave the rebels a wide berth.

At the office, we centrifuged the blood and prepared it for shipping. We sealed the package in three layers of plastic bags, absorbent newspapers, then a cardboard box. To be absolutely sure, we put that in a bigger box. Our package was the size of a medium-sized dog by the time Betsy and Conchy drove it to the airport.

We'd carefully labeled it with the words "Diagnostic Specimen" in big letters on two sides so the airline would take good care of it. The next day, the coup attempt ended.

I called Dr. Snow in Atlanta and told him to expect the samples the next day. But they didn't arrive. After three days, Budsy called the airline. "When it got to the US, they transferred it to American Airlines. American was short of planes, so they put it in an unrefrigerated warehouse in Texas. They plan to send it to Dr. Snow's lab tomorrow."

Of course, the lab found nothing.

Snow called to give me the bad news. "Look, Mark, I'm beginning to wonder if we're on the same team."

"How was I to know American would cook the package in Texas?

Justin said, "Things are looking up. I've got money for the travel budget. We'll send a team to do the study and collect specimens the right way."

"We'll need to get permission from the government first."

"I know. I already called the embassy. They tried, but your Secretary of Health said he'd have to talk to you first. Get to work."

The following day, I was in Dr. Bengzon's office. He was tall and leaned so far over his desk that he could bite me. "So, you tell me you already investigated the Ebola virus."

"Yes, sir."

"And you say the virus didn't make anyone sick."

"Yes."

"You know I'm in charge of negotiating the withdrawal of American troops from the Philippines."

"Yes, sir."

"Put yourself in my shoes, White. You've investigated, and nobody got sick. I've already asked the US to train our doctors to make a CDC here. How will it make me look if I still have to invite Americans to investigate because our doctors aren't good enough?"

"It's not that, sir. These people are experts. I'm sure they can teach us valuable lessons."

He drew himself up. "No, White, I won't have it."

I must have looked stricken because he uncharacteristically relented. "All right, I'll let them in, but there are conditions. They can't wear those spacesuits. If Filipinos wear paper gowns and masks, the Americans must do the same. And they can give no press conferences. They must slip in and out of the country so quietly that nobody knows they were here."

"Thank you, sir."

"I'm not finished. They can't ask the same questions your team did. They can't use our doctors and translators, either."

"Thank you so much, sir. I'm sure they'll do as you say."

I was elated. That night, I called Dr. Snow with the good news.

"Unacceptable," he declared. "We have to wear full protective gear. It's against the employee safety law to expose our employees to dangerous pathogens."

"But you said you used paper gowns against Ebola in Africa."

"That was before the law."

"The newspapers will pick up on you if you wear spacesuits."

"Can't be helped. I can agree not to make a statement. We will have to report to the Ambassador. I can't promise he won't give a presser."

"Do you plan to present your findings to Dr. Bengzon?"

"No."

I was getting worried. "He says you can't ask the same questions we did."

Snow said, "We'll have to. Your team, no disrespect, may have missed some subtle clues."

"Our team knows how to find subtle clues in Filipinos. I doubt yours can."

Of course, Dr. Bengzon refused them permission. But the CDC request had him thinking.

"White, if the media gets wind from CDC or anybody at the DOH that there is Ebola virus in the country, they will cry for our blood. We must tell them we've investigated and found no risk to public health. You and I are going to have a press conference this afternoon."

"But, sir, I'm an American."

"I regret that many of our people still have a colonial mentality. Also, if I go down because you gave me bad advice, I want to be sure you do, too."

"Can we have Betsy and Conchy there, too? They are the ones who did the study."

"Good idea," he said.

We did our best to make the press conference so dull that nobody would care. I was pleased to see every newspaper put the story on the back pages, where it rests in peace to this day.

CHAPTER 22
THE PISSING CONTEST

etsy and Conchy collected another set of samples from the monkeys. Sending samples to CDC failed, and they didn't seem to want to work with us. We needed a high-level safety lab to run our Ebola samples. Fast.

The US Naval Medical Research Unit-2 was a laboratory in Manila. They were famous for developing Oral Rehydration Solution (ORS). It saved millions of children and adults with cholera and other severe diarrheas. ORS replaces lost fluids and chemicals from severe diarrhea. It keeps the chemicals in the blood in good order and includes glucose to provide energy. It's still used all over the world. When I tried it, it tasted awful. Years later, when I got severe diarrhea, it tasted great. Everything is relative.

NAMRU-2 also had an excellent virology laboratory. Since CDC was so little help, I called the commander, Dr. Curtis Hayes.

He said, "We'd love to see if we can grow the viruses for you. Bring the specimens right over." They were a ten-minute walk from our office.

So we carried the precious little tubes across the San Lazaro compound and knocked on the door. Dr. Hayes came out to greet us. He was medium-build, brown-eyed, and wore a tan uniform. He gave us a tour of the little building. There were neat rooms for bacteria, viruses, and parasites.

Dr. Hayes carefully put the viruses in a biosafety box and said they'd have it on a jet to the US that day. Less than a week later, we got our first positives. I asked the navy to send some to CDC. I know he did this because Dr. Snow called me to complain.

I did send CDC the sera—the straw-colored fluid left after cells are removed from blood—from the healthy monkey handlers to see if they had antibodies. Three or four were positive, showing they'd been infected. None of their family members had been ill or had antibodies. This was more evidence that the gentle Asian strain of Ebola doesn't make people sick, let alone spread from person to person.

Finally, the nastygrams from Atlanta stopped, and I returned to my day job of teaching epidemiology and going to epidemics. Then I got a call from a friend at CDC.

"The new director of CDC started today."

"Thanks. Not sure this news merited a phone call to our fair island."

"His first act was to fire you."

"What? He doesn't even know my name."

The cheerful voice crackled across the wires. "He does now. The National Center for Infectious Diseases asked him to do it because you kept CDC personnel out of the Philippines."

"That's a bunch of shit. I moved heaven and earth to get them in. They insisted on wearing space suits and repeating our study. That was two no-gos for the Secretary of Health. Snow could have come anytime he wanted in regular clothes."

"Well, NCID called our office and asked us to tell you the bad news. You're fired."

"Is that why you're calling?"

"Of course not, you idiot. CDC can't hire people to work abroad. The State Department does that."

"And how does this help me?"

"USAID is part of State. We transferred you to USAID. You work for them."

"I get it." I laughed uneasily.

He snorted. "And everybody knows USAID hates CDC and all its works. They'll be pleased to stick a finger in CDC's eye by keeping you."

"You make these politics sound so evil and stupid."

"They are."

"Thanks for calling. You made my day."

"One last thing, stop sending emails about Ebola."

"Why?"

"The one you titled 'Ebolagate' riled everybody up."

"Who copied that to NCID?"

"Probably somebody who thought it was funny." He hung up.

Listening to the dial tone, I thought it was probably him.

The Ebolagate email *was* funny. It described NCID's floundering efforts to pressure me into bringing Dr. Snow and his team to Manila.

I enjoyed a quiet week with Budsy, Manolet, and the trainees. Then my office phone rang. "Dr. White, I'd like to invite you to meet with me. I'm the science attaché at the US Embassy, and I was asked to interview you about your Ebola virus investigation."

"Sure, I'll be happy to brief you. I'm pleased to hear from you. I thought the embassy didn't know I existed."

"We do now. Bring copies of your pertinent emails."

Son of a bitch. He was investigating me.

It took a six-pack of San Miguel beer to get to sleep. The following day, I put on a formal barong Tagalog and drove to the US Embassy complex overlooking Manila Bay. The science attaché's office was upstairs in the vast consulate building.

I was surprised that the attaché was wearing an open white shirt. I saw he'd hung his tie on a chair. I suspected he'd taken it off to make me feel at home. It didn't.

He swept around his big desk and patted a chair next to him. Together we faced a mahogany conference table. I handed him the thick folder of emails.

He flipped through it and handed it back. "Dr. White, you have powerful enemies."

I noticed he'd artfully combed his salt-and-pepper hair into waves on the sides.

I wondered if he was one of my enemies. "So it seems. Who wants my ass or head or whatever?"

"All I can tell you is that somebody in Washington sent us a stern cable saying your behavior made you a danger to US-Philippine relations. It sounded to me like they wanted us to PNG you."

The abbreviation means "persona non grata." It means a country expels a foreign spy or an undesirable. I had no idea the US could PNG me from the Philippines.

His brown eyes twinkled. "Tell me the story, and maybe I can give you some advice."

I thought he would probably advise me to leave the country before they had to send the marines. I told him the story anyway. If they're going to hang me, it should be for something I really did.

When I finished, he smiled and leaned back. "I thought it was something like this. I'd say someone has a contact at the DC State office and asked them to screw you. I regret that this happens occasionally.

"I wear two hats. In addition to science, I handle helping American drug companies sell to the Philippines. I'm thinking of having an intimate party and inviting Dr.

Bengzon to meet some executives with a very reasonable offer to sell him some pharmaceuticals."

"I can't ask him, sir. He hates Americans, including me. His priority is to get rid of brand-name drugs and substitute generics so the poor can afford them."

He leaned back, "I thought so. Still, I had to offer."

"What about the investigation?"

"Don't worry. I'll send a short report saying you are a great asset."

We shook, and I wandered around until I could find the way out.

A week later, the attaché called me. "You really do have powerful enemies."

"Are you going to kick me out?"

"Of course not. I'll reword the report I already sent. Also, I'll let some of my contacts in DC know what's going on. This ain't right."

"Thanks again, sir."

"No need to call me 'sir.' It makes me feel old."

When I returned to DOH, I told Manolet about the embassy visit.

He looked appalled. "Come with me now. We're going to see Dr. Bengzon. He'll want to know right away."

As we stood before the secretary's desk, I couldn't control my shaking hands as I told the story.

When I finished talking, a grim smile was on Dr. Bengzon's face. "Mark, this is a clear intrusion into my department. I'll take care of it."

After we walked out of the office, Manolet laughed. "He called you Mark. I think he trusts you—the enemy of his enemy.

The next day, my friend in Atlanta called me.

"Holy shit, your Secretary of Health called the head of the Department of Health and Human Services. He told him he didn't care if DHHS allowed pissing contests to impair its efficiency, but Dr. Bengzon will not accept DHHS employees pissing on his department."

"Holy shit."

"Yes, holy shit. CDC fired Snow—and his girlfriend for good measure. Please ask Dr. Bengzon to give us a time for the director of NCID to meet him in Manila to apologize."

"OK."

A week later, Jim Hughes, NCID director, arrived at my office for an 8:00 a.m. appointment.

I walked him across the compound to the secretary's office. We sat there for an hour. Then an assistant told us Dr. Bengzon had some urgent business and would meet us at 6:00 p.m.

Hughes, a mensch notwithstanding his baying for my blood, told many jokes in the morning, then spent the day napping on my couch.

At six, the assistants told us we would be in soon. As the hours passed, Jim got understandably crabby. I was crabby myself.

At eight, we were ushered into the secretary's office. He did not shake Jim's hand. We stood facing him across the great desk.

"Dr. Hughes, Dr. White is the most valuable consultant I have. He's helped us share information and ideas with many of CDC's programs. If you pull him out, rest assured we will pull out of arrangements with your government, including the immunization and diarrheal disease programs."

"I understand, sir. We fired the person who caused the trouble, and I assure you it'll never happen again."

"It better not," Dr. Bengzon said. He turned his attention to the stack of papers on his desk.

We realized we were dismissed.

Once the craziness was over, Betsy wrote an excellent paper telling the world we'd discovered a new mild variant of the Ebola virus. This was big news since it might lead to a vaccine. There was only a small, tight-knit group of scientists working on Ebola in the US, and they were all friends. We feared Snow would block us from publishing in an American journal. So Betsy and I submitted it to the prestigious British journal, the *Lancet*.

The editor soon emailed back. "The reviewers I consulted said it didn't belong in a general medical journal. I think it is of interest, so I'm offering to publish it as a letter to the editor. I'm sure you'll want to send it somewhere else."

Betsy emailed back, "We'd be honored to be published in your letters section."

There followed hours of tooth-gnashing editing to shrink our full-length article to fit the letter word limit. When we finished, all the essential facts were there. It was concise and readable.

It was duly published.

I thought it would be my claim to fame if I ever investigated an Ebola epidemic. But our Asian strain was mild. Not like headline news stories from Africa, where hospitals overflowed with people with raging fevers bleeding to death as horrified doctors and nurses helplessly looked on.

Just my bad luck, I guess.

I could have been a contender.

CHAPTER 23

THE HUNCHBACK OF NOTRE DAME

My newfound visibility at the embassy paid off a few months later when they invited us to their Christmas party. As I dressed, I watched Budsy's silhouette in the steamy shower curtain. Then she reached out and took my hand. "I've got a breast lump." She guided my hand to her small left breast. My fingers felt a hard, sharp-edged mass about two centimeters across. It felt like cancer. The only good thing was that it wasn't attached to her chest wall.

She stood naked, rivulets of water pouring down her skin, looking up at me. I said, "We'd better see the doctor tomorrow."

"Yes," she said and turned to towel herself off.

I was stunned. A bottomless ache opened up in my chest, and the world stopped. I realized I had been standing still the entire time she dried off. She nudged me. "Time to finish dressing for the Year's Eve party."

I'd seen her like this before. In her many years as head nurse and supervisor for intensive care units, no matter what the crisis, she knew what to do. She'd calmly disappear into the closet where she stashed an extra crash set or run down to the pharmacy and intimidate a recalcitrant pharmacist into giving her the drug we needed to save a life. In quiet times, she could be crabby and fly into rages, but that was for show. The real Budsy was the calm, competent one.

We had a surprisingly good time at the party.

On January second, we were in the office of the leading breast surgeon in Manila. He dressed immaculately. He had long, sensitive fingers—the kind you want to see on your surgeon. The next day, I met him outside the operating room. He stood tall, with firm muscles filling the sleeves and chest of his scrubs. They were in the OR for about twenty minutes. Then a nurse led me to Budsy in the recovery room and left on some errand. It broke my heart to see her in the cart, woozily staring up over the raised sides. I cried and petted her head. Her hair was soaked with sweat. She didn't speak. Then she began to squirm and reach through the bars, waving her arm. "Falling," she said.

"You're not falling. It's the drugs. They'll wear off soon."

"Not me, you bonehead, the guy behind you."

I turned to see the only other patient in the room climbing over the rails of his cart, on the verge of a nasty fall.

Budsy grabbed my arm as I turned to settle him down. She reached through his bars and soothed him.

The door swung open, and our surgeon signaled me to come out. "It's cancer. You'll need to tell her." So much for our macho stud muffin doctor. "I didn't see any spread to the chest walls or lymphatics. It's probably one point nine centimeters in diameter." The size of breast lumps is essential because it predicts how malignant they will be—and how long you will probably live. Budsy, who had spent several years in an oncology practice caring for cancer patients, knew this and a great deal more about what happens to treat cancer patients.

I went back to her. She looked up at my face. "It's malignant," she said. Of course, we'd both expected cancer the moment we felt the mass.

"How big?"

"One point nine centimeters."

If a lump is two centimeters or more, you can improve your chances of survival by taking chemotherapy and radiotherapy.

She exhaled and coughed. "Whew, I don't have to have chemo and radiation." It was a close call.

I said, "Thank God. I'll get you some ice chips for your throat."

We decided to be on the safe side and have her breast removed. Since we'd worked together at Booth Memorial Medical Center in Queens, New York, we flew back to see our friends in the surgery department. She chose Kenny Rifkind, a scholarly general surgeon. He was balding with dark red hair and deep, sympathetic eyes. His secretary set us up with appointments with specialists to help us decide on the treatment plan.

Everybody with breast cancer faces important and painful choices. Does she want reconstructive surgery to replace the breast with fat from elsewhere on her body or with a bag of silicone? What about radiotherapy and chemotherapy?

The medical literature provides guidance on many decisions, but the science is unclear for others. And things like the choice of a prosthesis are esthetic choices. The specialist I remember best was the plastic surgeon, Dr. Godfrey. We both knew him. His large office was on Park Avenue. We moved through three waiting rooms, each more intimate than the one before. Tasteful original art covered the walls. One featured a rosy, Rubenesque lady staring provocatively into the eyes of the viewer. There was also a Modigliani nude, cool, lithe, and sultry. The sculptures were similar. Smooth white planes and curves that begged to be stroked. Dr. Godfrey was a sculptor of the difficult medium of human flesh.

The ambiance was calm and unhurried, everything in superb taste. You needn't ask how much your surgery would cost. Plenty. As we glided through the rooms and corridors, I envied the surgeon and wished I'd been able to take his path. We could see he was respected, loved, and rich.

The doctor rose to greet us in his inner sanctum, hugging Buds. "I follow your adventures in the Philippines. You are saving so many lives and preventing so much suffering. If only I could be like you." I had to stifle the urge to offer to trade. The grass is always greener.

He asked Budsy to remove her top and appraised her rounded, small breasts. He ran long, sensitive fingers lightly over the surface, reading the texture and warmth—a connoisseur.

In the end, she decided against plastic surgery. "If you love me, you'll love me with one breast."

"I do, and I will."

She chose against chemotherapy. She'd been an oncology nurse and knew the pros and cons. Especially the cons.

Our job at the Philippine DOH was finally ending, but WHO hired me to return to the Philippines with Budsy to do HIV surveillance and control. She threw herself into the job. Most cases were in what was politely called "female commercial sex workers" or FCSW.

While prostitution was illegal, the health department could best control the spread of venereal diseases by teaching the women about safe sex. They treated them when they got sick and traced their customers to treat them and stop the spread.

In each business, Budsy gathered the FCSW in a big room. "Ladies," she'd announce, "condoms are your best friends. They keep you from getting sick or pregnant."

Usually, someone would ask, "What do we do if the customer doesn't want to wear a condom?"

Budsy would smile. "I thought you might ask that." She bought an ashtray with a gross wooden dildo sticking up. She would put the condom in her teeth and slide it onto the dildo.

Then she supervised each woman as they practiced putting condoms on with their mouths. She gained enough notoriety that the Archbishop of Cebu showed up at one of her courses and threatened to excommunicate her. She was incensed, even though she hadn't been to church in decades.

A year or so later, her doctor gave her some follow-up X-rays and found a lump in the right upper lobe of her lung. It was a recurrence of her breast cancer. We immediately made reservations to fly to New York and our surgical friends.

This time we saw Tretorn Pugham, a slight and wiry Thai thoracic surgeon. He drove a Ferrari and would occasionally race other doctors. Once, I challenged him to a race with my Chrysler Laser.

He smiled benignly. "If you can beat that cardiologist in his 240z, I'll take you on," he said.

These races were dangerous because they were on the Long Island Expressway in the middle of the night. I never challenged the cardiologist, so I spared myself the humiliation of being crushed.

Tretorn told Budsy, "I agree the mass is worrisome. It sits in the center of the right upper lobe, which makes it very hard to biopsy without opening you up. I'll take you to the OR and do the open biopsy day after tomorrow. We'll have to take the lobe if the frozen section is positive. You can live without a right upper lobe."

"OK," she said. I saw a flicker of fear in her eyes.

The next day, Budsy seemed relaxed and calm. She paced a while, then sat looking calmly into the distance.

When we got to the hospital, she filled out all the forms with an odd little smile. A nurse started her IVs. As they wheeled her through the big double doors to the OR, she raised her hand and waved to me.

I was nervous and went for a walk around the hospital. My favorite floors were those with the ICUs, so I headed up there. The head of the medical ICU was a good friend. His name was Mel Hochman, a quintessential New Yorker. Tall and balding with a gray-black wreath of hair around his head, he loved to joke. I've always thought people in stressful jobs need a good sense of humor to avoid being overwhelmed by the tragedy around them. It was impossible not to like Mel's sharp wit.

I heard my name on the PA system and ran up the stairs to the OR suite. It was no surprise when Tretorn told me the mass was cancer and he'd taken the lobe.

Budsy lay unconscious in the recovery room, on a respirator with a noisy chest tube sucking out fluid and air from around the rest of her lung. When she opened her eyes, I leaned down over and kissed her. She was stable.

A cloud of exhaustion engulfed me. I walked down to the surgical on-call rooms and found an empty room and bed. The next day, they removed Budsy's endotracheal tube. Tretorn transferred her and her noisy chest tube to a private room, where she spent several days. She was hoarse and coughed a lot, but we were profoundly thankful she'd gotten through the stress and was OK. There was a lounge chair, but it was hard to sleep with the noise, so I often paced the nursing floors or slept in on-call rooms. Sometimes a nurse would grab my arm and tell me visiting hours were long over. Then another would say, "He's Dr. White. He used to work here. His wife is in the ICU." Then they'd leave me alone.

For showers, I'd go to the dressing rooms outside the ORs.

All this nocturnal wandering down dark corridors made me feel like the Hunchback of Notre Dame.

CHAPTER 24
STEM CELLS

O nce Budsy recovered from her surgery, she wanted the most powerful available chemotherapy. At the time, an experimental treatment called stem-cell transplant looked promising. Fortunately, my brother-in-law, Mark Campbell, was an oncologist and agreed to give Budsy a stem cell treatment for cancer, off protocol. He was not doing it as part of his formal research.

We flew to my sister's house in Grand Rapids, Michigan, and he evaluated her to see if she could handle the powerful therapy. He decided she could. She passed all the tests with flying colors. We flew back to our apartment in Manila to rest and take the grueling chemotherapy needed before the transplant began.

Budsy's oncologist in Manila agreed to prescribe the drugs. We bought them at the hospital pharmacy and brought the IV bags and ampoules of medicines home. Her nephew made a wooden IV pole. She would sit in an easy chair as I started an IV and gave her the drugs. The nastiest was Adriamycin, a bright orange liquid. It looked evil, but she never had a bad reaction. "When I was an oncology nurse," she said, leaning back, "we used to call this Killer Kool-Aid."

In Grand Rapids, we stayed in my sister's large rambling

house. They were generous in welcoming us. Mark was a highly successful entrepreneur who owned several used and new car lots and huge oncology practice. He had been touched by cancer himself. When he got prostate cancer, he must have made a bucket list because he bought a Harley Davidson dealership and took to riding a big one. In addition to being a risk-taker, Mark was a superb manager, thoughtful of his staff and patients, and always looking for ways to improve their treatment and lives.

Mark has a steady hand and calm brown eyes. We witnessed this firsthand when he did a bone marrow biopsy on Budsy. Mark had her lay on her side, then drove a huge trocar—a hollow tube with a very sharp end—into her pelvic bone, twisting and leaning on it before sucking back to harvest a large quantity of marrow. Budsy stiffened, her eyes bulged, and tears ran down her face as she looked at the huge syringe half-full of dark-red marrow.

Afterward, Mark said, "Budsy, are we still friends?" I feared she would say no, but she shook her head yes.

He said, "Here's what happens next. Breast cancer is unpredictable. Some cancers, even big ones, may be firm and not shed cells. The surgery may have cured you. But some-times, even small tumors shed thousands of malignant cells into the bloodstream. The cells can land anywhere and start new tumors.

"The problem is we can't tell which, so I think it's safest to treat the blood." Mark stood in his white coat, looking us straight in the eye as he talked. His calm demeanor and competence made us feel good as we entered the dangerous new world.

"Your bone marrow makes blood cells, including stem cells. When your body needs to make a new kind of cells, the stem cells grow into that kind of cells. It's amazing.

"We'll take your bone marrow and isolate the white cells, including the stem cells. We freeze these."

Mark took a long breath. "Now that we have a backup, we treat you with extremely high doses of chemotherapy—enough to kill the rest of your bone marrow and—we hope—any cancer cells."

Budsy was sick as a dog on the high-dose chemotherapy, but she got through it.

Our next visit to Mark's office was the big one. Mark's assistant, a young nurse named Matt, ushered us into a room where she lay on a big, padded table. He asked what music she liked. "I'll make enough music myself, thank you," she said. Next, Mark came in with a little plastic bag containing the treated cells from Budsy's biopsy. That bag was her only passport to survival.

"The blood is cold, so we'll heat it on the way in, but it's often still chilly. There are blankets near the bed.

"To prevent the blood clotting in the bag, we take away the calcium. When the decalcified blood goes back in, it will suck all the calcium out of your body, so we need to replace it as quickly as possible."

He took a giant bottle of Tums from a shelf. "They're made of calcium. Try to take a few every minute. We get mixed flavors to make it easier. Be sure to chew them."

Budsy's face turned gray.

"There's a bowl here just in case you feel nauseous." She looked ill already. So did I.

Matt hung the blood bag, and Mark opened the valve a little. You could see the blood run slowly down the transparent tube. As it reached her arm, she shivered. "Check her blood pressure and pulse, Matt.

"Of course, you can get allergic reactions like anaphylaxis with the cells, just like any other blood product."

Her blood pressure was fine, and Mark strode out of the room. Budsy popped a couple of Tums in her mouth, chewed, and swallowed. She made a face.

"Buds, you mixed red and green. Maybe you'll do better if you stick to one color at a time."

She looked at me coolly. "Get me a couple of blankets."

I lay the blankets on top of her. Then I sat down, a book in my lap. I never looked at it. I watched her every second of the four hours of the infusion. She didn't like it, but she took it uncomplainingly.

I drove her home that night and helped her to bed. My sister Marty Jo was waiting for us at the door. "I'd ask you how you feel, but I think I already know."

She was right. All the chemotherapy and Tums had left her nauseous. Marty Jo, a nurse herself, hovered, soothing Budsy, taking her vital signs and making her comfortable. I paced the house for hours, and every time I checked, Buds was sleeping fitfully. I got to sleep near dawn, just after Mark came home. He worked like a dog, far into the night, then got up after two or three hours to head back to make his morning rounds on his patients in the hospital. He didn't make all that money through good luck.

For the next three days, Marty Jo sat with us. We could barely get enough water, juice, and ice cream down Budsy to stave off dehydration. Then one morning, she rolled over and poked me. "I'm hungry."

"That's great. What shall I make?"

"I'm craving lobster heads. Get me lobster heads."

That seemed a good idea. I'd get a couple of lobsters and boil them up. Budsy would eat the heads, and I'd get the claws and tails—a marriage made in heaven.

We'd slept through a power outage that night. In every grocery store I visited, the story was the same. The air pumps in the lobster tanks had been off, and the lobsters were all dead. I had to drive to the neighboring town of Muskegon before I found a store with live lobsters. I realized I hadn't had breakfast and was starving. I rushed back to the house, breaking a few speeding laws and bending others.

The kitchen was far from our room, and Budsy kept me busy ordering me to add the right spices. They made our lobsters succulent and tender. She slowly ate the two heads. I feasted on one of the tails and put the other in the refrigerator. Marty Jo's son Scott ate the other when he got home from school.

As she got better, we moved to stay with my brother Thomas and his wife, Sibyl, in their big white farmhouse in Saint Johns, famous for its mint farms. I think one of their daughters was chosen to be Mint Queen once. Thomas and Sibyl were wonderful. Years later, he had a near-fatal heart attack and had emergency surgery in Honolulu. He said his Filipina nurse made him feel that Budsy, competent and nurturing, was helping pull him through.

As she got better, I took her to Traverse City. It's up at the top of the lower peninsula in Cherry County. The annual Cherry Festival was going on. We ate tons of cherries every day. The tart sweetness of cherries exploding in my mouth reminded me of the intense pleasure of life.

I was pleased to see the Cherry County Playhouse was still there. When I was sixteen, my family vacationed at the Cherry Festival, and the Cherry County Playhouse was opposite our hotel. It was in a big yellowish tent. It was a star system theater, which meant they always had a star from TV or movies doing summer stock there. I liked theater and had done a lot of drama in high school. They began to recognize me as I showed up for production after production. A guy came up to me and invited me to be an apprentice there. I couldn't believe my luck. Neither could my parents, who swiftly agreed to let me spend the rest of the summer there.

The work was insanely hard. Before a new show, we'd be up all night. I helped Chris, the sound man, make tapes with all the cues. He had a pile of records with sound effects. We'd record them and then splice white leader tape between them to get the sounds right. If there was no record of the sound we needed, we would make it and tape it. Great fun.

After each show, we'd "police the theater," meaning pick up all the trash. The professional actors took us to a bar a couple of nights a week. The bartender would let us in the back to a private room, where we'd all drink beers and have a terrific time. One night, the bartender came in and said, "The bulls, get out of here." He meant the police. We rushed laughing out into the night. Good times.

And we acted. I played the twenty-third sailor in *South Pacific*. I had a line, too. It was either "Yes" or "No."

My only starring role was in the kids' shows. I played Candlewick, the evil boy who leads Pinocchio astray. The kids were a great audience. After the performances, they'd ask us to autograph programs. It's the only time in my life anybody asked for my autograph.

I shared these reminiscences with Budsy. "That explains a lot," she said.

My contract in the Philippines ended while we were in the US, and an acquaintance offered me a job where we could rest and regain our strength. It was in Kampala, Uganda.

CHAPTER 25

THE WHITE LADY AND THE RED LADY

he guy who offered me the job was Seth Berkely, another CDC alumnus. He described the situation in Uganda. "Here's the deal: A few months after rebels led by Yoweri Museveni ousted Idi Amin and the corrupt leaders who followed, Jimmy Carter hired me to work for his foundation to help rebuild the Ugandan Ministry of Health."

Seth did an excellent job for Jimmy's foundation, and the Rockefeller Foundation, impressed by his work, hired him to supervise health projects from their New York City office. He proposed hiring me to create an epidemiology training program that combined the strengths of the FETPs and Schools of Public Health. He called it by the snappy name of Public Health School Without Walls, pronounced P-H-S-WOW.

I was quick to take Seth up on his offer. He flew Budsy and me to Kampala for a job interview.

After a long flight, we arrived at Entebbe Airport on the shores of Lake Victoria. As we circled, I scanned the lake for the source of the Nile but didn't see it. Off the edge of the runway sat the burned-out remains of some fighter jets. Palestinian terrorists highjacked an Air France flight from Paris to Israel. Israeli commandos rescued the hostages and blew up the Ugandan fighters to cover their escape. This happened years ago, but it looked as if it happened yesterday.

At Customs, two big men in double-breasted suits took us out of line and deposited us in a windowless basement room for interrogation. There were rusting filing cabinets along the walls. We tried to step around papers lying on the floor in the dim light, many decorated with colorful stamps. Another tall, thin man in a worn uniform walked in and fired questions. He periodically flew into what seemed to be dangerous rages. Thinking he wanted a bribe, I tried to remember how much money was in my wallet. I hoped he'd take dollars.

Suddenly the door flew open and slammed against the wall. An older man stuck his head in and said, "*Eeeee*, this man is for Bukenya." Ugandans use "eeeee" to express alarm and concern. Whoever he was, this Bukenya was an important man. A lot of Swahili followed, and the customs man eventually led us out of the building to a dark parking lot in the back. He watched us step into the darkness. I'll never forget the feeling of his baleful eye on my back before he closed the door. We walked quickly out among the lines of cars.

Nobody arrested us, nobody tried to mug us, but nobody offered to help us, either. Mosquitoes buzzed in our ears. The ones that bite at night can give you malaria. We heard night-birds. What we didn't hear or see were taxis or buses to Kampala. Even though Idi Amin was long gone, I thought about how his soldiers disappeared thousands of people.

A vehicle turned down our row, and its bright headlights pinned us back against the door. Then the car honked. My legs felt shaky as I walked around the lights to the driver's side.

"Professor Bukenya sent me. My name is John," the driver, a pleasant middle-aged man, said.

Budsy and I got in the back seat. It was about fifty miles to our hotel, the Fairview in Kampala, and John sped down the road. I later learned bandits hide by roads and roll logs out to stop your car. People advised us to drive fast and evasively. John took this advice to heart.

We arrived in good order. Budsy instantly fell asleep in our room, but I tossed and turned, worrying about the next day's interview. She looked so soft as she slept, and a faint smile was on her lips. Her ladylike snores kept me awake, but I finally drifted off. Then a brassy Congolese band began playing on the terrace below us. I was ready to give up.

At about 9:00 p.m., a waiter from the open-air bar below knocked on the door. I'd wrapped my head up in pillows, so he had to bang a couple of times.

"Go away," I snarled at him.

"Sir, Professor Bukenya wants you to join him."

So this was the famous Bukenya. I'd have to go.

"Tell him I'll be right down."

I went to the bathroom and washed my face. I tried to do my chest and armpits, hoping to smell less sweaty. I said, "Buds, I'll be gone for a few minutes."

She may have heard since she rolled over.

I walked down to the open-air bar. A waiter led me to a table where Professor Bukenya, a large black man, looked up. The jacket of his double-breasted suit hung on the back of his chair.

He stood halfway up and waved me to the only vacant chair. "Sit down, White." He smiled at the big, red-faced white man sitting across from us. "This is Bill Bertrand, Vice President for International Health at Tulane University."

Bill waved a big bottle of Nile Special beer at me in a toasting motion. He, too, wore a suit. You could see his big biceps through his coat sleeves. His shirt buttons gaped over his chest. I later learned he was an ex-marine. Most people called him Wild Bill Bertrand, a name he richly deserved. Bill said, "Professor Gilbert Bukenya is head of the Makerere School of Public Health."

"Hey, my brother," Gilbert shouted at a waiter. Bring this man a beer. Bring us all a beer." The waiter nodded and disappeared. Gilbert and Wild Bill had already finished at least one bottle before I arrived.

"My brother, bring us some goat," Gilbert shouted again. Ten minutes later, somebody brought skewers of delicious, barbecued goat.

Wild Bill pointed at my nearly empty bottle. Professor Bukenya reached out and grabbed the arm of a passing server. "A bottle of red lady and one of white lady. Three glasses, too."

The red and white ladies turned out to be wine. We talked over the band, but I can't remember what we discussed—certainly not epidemiology training.

After the wine and goat course, my hosts ordered a bottle of Scotch. "No thanks, guys," I croaked. "Scotch tastes of burlap bags to me. How about bourbon?"

They didn't have bourbon, so the professor ordered a bottle of VSOP Cognac.

"No worry about the cost," he said, patting my shoulder heavily. "Rockefeller's paying, and I'm taking leftovers home."

I listened to Bukenya and Wild Bill talk as if I were rolled up in a thick carpet. They seemed to be having a great time, but my brain and tongue were seriously furry.

Finally, I ventured, "Guys, you've made me feel welcome, but I need to get some sleep before my interview tomorrow."

Wild Bill said, "The interview is over."

"What?"

Professor Bukenya said, "Call me Gilbert." He pulled my curriculum vitae from his pocket and opened it to the page that listed my publications. "You list over thirty publications, but only three have your name as the first author."

"Is that good?"

"Splendid. Your students are first authors, so they get full credit for their work and a good start for their careers. That's priceless. Not many consultants do that."

"So, am I hired?"

"We hired you before you left Manila. Have another brandy."

I stumbled back to my room before the world got too tippy.

Three months later, Budsy and I returned to Uganda to start work. In Manila, the US Embassy had put us in a large house in a safe neighborhood. Things were different in Kampala. Budsy and I were not affiliated with the US Embassy, and they didn't provide housing or protection—or anything else. The tiny US "embassy" was a few rented rooms in the back of the British High Commission. The few times I heard the US ambassador speak, he emphasized that Uganda was of no strategic importance to the US and that his job was primarily to provide humanitarian aid. When I later visited the USAID office, they told me not to ask for money for the training program because they didn't see the utility of epidemiology in general and our project in particular. So there.

On our first night in Kampala, Gilbert made us reservations in the towering Sheraton Hotel, the tallest building in Kampala. We could see dozens of birds sailing over the town from our lofty balcony. They circled in three layers. Songbirds made up the lowest level. The next was hideous Maribu storks, large dirty, ungainly refuse-eaters. Their bills looked and sounded like wood when they snapped them, as they often did. Above them soared the vultures. I once walked down a side street and came upon a group of them, beaks red with gore, devouring a dead dog.

Gilbert helped us immensely. He found us a wonderful house in a development called Ministers' Village in the suburb of Ntinda. We were pleased that he and his lovely wife, Margaret, lived a few blocks away.

He had also hired two twenty-four-hour security guards, which seemed like an unnecessary expense. "You'll need the guards in case of petty criminals," Gilbert told us.

Budsy eyed him. "What petty crimes are we talking about?"

"A gang of thieves backs a moving van up to your house and takes all the furniture and everything else."

Budsy took a breath. "If that's a petty crime, what's a regular crime?"

"They kidnap you, too."

CHAPTER 26
DR. SMITH, I PRESUME

Our new house was made of brownish bricks with a veranda where we would sit and look over the broken glass atop our fence down the hills at the lush green landscape shambling down the slope.

At sunset the first night, we heard rifle shots and the occasional burps of automatic weapons and explosions that might have been grenades or bombs. There was a curfew. Starting from 6:00 p.m., soldiers fired on anybody they saw. Some people fired back. This was much worse than the coup attempts in the Philippines.

I went out to consult the guards but found they had loosed two vicious dogs that rushed around between the house and the wall, snarling and barking. We lay awake, gnawing fear never far away. It turned out this was a typical night.

In the morning, we unlocked the barred door to our bedroom and the entrance to the outside so our cook and maid could come in. Our landlady had arranged for two young women from her home village to be our maid and cook. Also, there was Gerald, an alcoholic young man who did odd jobs and kept the dogs. We learned that dogs and cats are not so much pets as work animals that protect people from thieves and rats.

Ugandans euphemistically referred to the nightly shooting as "a bit of a peace and order problem." Gilbert, it turned out, had been active in the resistance, and Museveni knew and trusted him. Later he would name Gilbert vice president. Probably this explained Gilbert's power and the universal respect—and sometimes fear—people showed when anyone mentioned his name.

Our diet featured daily servings of *matoke*, pronounced *mato-kay*, the Ugandan national food. Matoke is mostly fiber, and Ugandans have the highest fiber diets in the world. They made it of steamed green bananas, a bland canvas to flavor with fish, meat, peanut sauce, etc. To get enough nourishment, you must eat a pile of matoke the size of your head with each meal.

Toilets have to be huge to handle the load.

East Africans count time differently from Westerners. One o'clock starts at daybreak, 6:00 a.m. Western time, and so on. When you think about it, starting the count in the morning makes more sense than starting in the middle of the night.

Not long after we moved into our new house, we were eating a breakfast of matoke and eggs when there was a knock on the gate. Gerald let in a tall man wearing a bright traditional shirt, blue jeans, and leather sandals. His short hair was streaked with gray.

His voice was low and sonorous. "Greetings and welcome to the neighborhood. I am your resistance chairman. You can call me RC."

"Resistance against what?" asked Budsy, ever the skeptic.

"I was a soldier in Museveni's rebel army. When we captured an area, the army organized the people and left them with an organizational structure before moving on. Because I come from this neighborhood, the people chose me as the resistance chairman. The revolution's been over for a few years, but the RC system remains."

"Nice to meet you, sir," I said.

"My house is just down the street, at the corner there. Call on me if there is anything you need."

Budsy eyed him. "Like what?"

The chairman laughed that deep and hearty African laugh. "You'll know it when you see it. Also, it is my duty to collect revolutionary taxes."

I was ready to call Gilbert to intercede before this stranger conned us.

"The tax is ten thousand shillings."

Since ten thousand shillings was ten dollars, we paid him off, and he left, undoubtedly to spread joy to our neighbors. We would meet the RC again and learn our taxes were a good investment.

Seth visited Kampala every few months to check on the program, often accompanied by a female graduate student. He'd take us to dinner at the fancy Fang Fang Chinese restaurant and tell the story of how his Ugandan girlfriend had left him. Women loved Seth, and he loved them back.

One evening, he brought a graduate student named Bernadette. She had long brown hair and wore jeans, a white blouse with a Peter Pan collar, and a red slash of lipstick.

Seth told us his Ugandan girlfriend left him. "I'm still broken up," Seth said. He showed us a picture of an attractive black woman. "That woman was the world to me."

Budsy nudged me. "He's a love 'em and leave 'em, a womanizer. Fat chance she broke up with him."

Seth's eyes seemed unfocused. "I travel as much as possible rather than stay in my empty apartment in Manhattan. Every night I make a simple French dinner, light a candle, put on some quiet music, and imagine her across the table."

The grad student's eyes seemed to be tearing up.

Budsy whispered loudly, "Not a dry lap in the house."

Mortified, I hissed, "For God's sake, shut the fuck up, Buds."

Conversation stopped. Everyone looked at me. Seth put down his drink, and I thought I saw a little smile on his lips.

The university provided me with a white four-wheel-drive Suzuki Vitara to get to work. One day as I drove toward the university, the engine fell out over a railroad track. It was easy to hitch a ride to the city, and I later learned that Gilbert had sent the car for a tune-up to make it ready for us. The mechanics had replaced only two of the six screws that held the engine. They'd kept the other four for later use. There was corruption—even down to screws—like the mechanics who stole our lug nuts in the Philippines. Once the mechanics put all the screws in, the Vitara worked faithfully for the rest of my time there.

My office was a hike up to the fourth floor, next to Gilbert's. Budsy, still recovering from the stem cell transplant to treat her recurrent breast cancer, struggled with the stairs. She spent most of the days resting on the couch in my office and helping with the myriad of office work.

In contrast to the embassy and USAID, people at the medical school were excited by the program. This was a problem since it was the custom for each department chairman to name two students to be admitted to other departments. We only had room for twelve doctors, who needed to be highly competent and dedicated. The department chairs' nominees were neither, so the tradition was a threat.

A typical interview began with a satisfied young man leaning back comfortably in his chair.

I'd ask, "Why do you want to study field epidemiology?"

"Sounds interesting."

"Why?"

"The dean of my college told me so. He said you'd understand."

After the first interview, Gilbert told me, "Sorry, White. This is a strong custom, and I can't piss off all the other department heads."

That night, Gilbert, Wild Bill, and I went drinking.

As we sipped our first round of Nile Specials, I said, "Bill, we're in trouble."

He took a slug of beer and raised an eyebrow. "So soon? What happened?

Gilbert and I rushed to tell our story.

Wild Bill laughed. "I can't believe you don't know this, Gilbert. Happens to universities all the time."

Gilbert stiffened.

I leaned in for a reassuring handful of groundnuts, as they call peanuts in Africa. "So tell us, Bill, what's the solution?"

He smiled. "Simple. You make the tuition so high that nobody can afford it. Then you offer scholarships to the applicants you want."

Gilbert and I raised the tuition to ridiculous levels, higher than the famous London School of Hygiene and Tropical Medicine. Then we accepted all the students who applied, including the legacies from the other departments. It didn't matter since none of them could pay the tuition. We were surprised that a passionate young health educator sold his house and car to pay tuition. We liked his attitude and quietly gave him a scholarship, too. He turned out to be one of our most successful graduates.

Faculty meetings usually took place in restaurants. The first was in a little bar in town. We ordered drinks and snacks, and then Gilbert read each agenda item from a list he'd scribbled on a napkin. Of course, Gilbert sat at the head of the table and the rest of us along the sides.

"First," he said in his deep, growly voice, "in the future, I will have complete control of all funds coming into any research projects in the School of Public Health."

David Serwadda, who had hundreds of thousands of

dollars in grants from the US NIH to do AIDS research, stood. "Gilbert, I can't be responsible for my grant funding if you can veto me or dip into my money."

Gilbert stood, too. "I've had a letter from the NIH about you. They mentioned your grant as an example. They reminded me that I am responsible for all their grants to the school and that I must personally vouch for them. Otherwise, they may not continue to fund our projects. I must insist."

Serwadda stood his ground, fists, and jaw clenched.

Gilbert focused his small, red eyes on Serwadda. An interminable second or two passed until Serwadda looked away.

"Unless there are more objections, I'll record this as unanimous." No one spoke. Gilbert sat, called for another round, and went on to his next priority.

Professor Ndugutsi said, "If you're going to be that way, the least you can do is pay for the beer." It was a sensible proposal.

"I'm here to serve," Gilbert said with a gracious nod. The rest of the meeting ran smoothly, with toasts after each of the so-called votes.

I sat next to Fred Wabire, an intelligent young professor who'd gotten his Ph.D. from Johns Hopkins. When I excused myself by saying I had to pee, he whispered, "You don't say that in our country. Tell people, 'I have to make a phone call.'"

I thanked him for this cultural education. He smiled back. "If you have to defecate, say, 'I need to make a long-distance call.'"

I should have known he was teasing. After the beer, I soon needed to pee. When I rose to "make a phone call," he handed me his cell phone. Everybody laughed—initiation over.

The following day, Budsy and I climbed the stairs to my office. We heard scrabbling and skittering as we reached the fourth floor and opened the door. A troupe of long-tailed black monkeys with whitish bellies rushed down the hall, bouncing off each other and the walls. They looked guilty as sin, of course, because they were. They surged out the fire entrance, where somebody had left the door unlocked. We watched them tumbling and chittering down and into the trees.

I met the students in a friendly classroom. It had actual blackboards, and for the only time in years of teaching, I left with chalk on my hands, pants, and shoes each day. I've always disliked the whiteboard markers since I can taste the bitter solvent on my tongue. If that gets into my bloodstream, what effects might it have? Anyway, the chalk period was a happy one.

I had asked different professors to teach classes with me, but all made excuses except for Bazeo, the occupational medicine professor. He always started with the father of occupational medicine, the eminent Bernardino Ramazzini, who lived in the seventeenth century.

So I had to present nearly all the classes. This wasn't as hard as it might seem. The morning was lectures and short problems. I had notes for all my lessons from the Philippines and case studies I had taught them for seven years. Each afternoon was a single large case study that trainees worked on together. They worked except for when students burst into laughter when they figured out that the food that caused the epidemic was fish balls. You can imagine the cries of "They eat fish's balls there?"

I was troubled that only one professor would teach with me, and for once, Gilbert didn't seem able to help.

One afternoon when the trainees were working on a long case study, I strolled around the building. I looked in an open office door and saw a tall gentleman with salt-and-pepper hair working at a computer.

I said, "Hi, I'm the new training director for the MPH program in the P-H-S-WOW."

"Nice to meet you," he said in a mellifluous English

accent. "I'm Peter Smith, from the London School of Hygiene and Tropical Medicine."

"Cool."

Peter seemed to startle and raised a white eyebrow above brown eyes that shone with intelligence. "I teach statistics. I'm head of the Biostatistics Department at the London School of Hygiene and Tropical Medicine. I'm here on sabbatical, hoping to help teach the students and do a little AIDS research."

"You must be very busy. Teaching loads must be heavy. There are lots of students here. Mine certainly is."

"I am only supervising the thesis of one Ph.D. student. I'd hoped to be more helpful." He paused. "I'm rewriting one of my books, and they send me things from London, so I'm busy." He seemed a bit defensive.

I saw my chance. "Only one Ugandan has agreed to teach in the MPH program. The rest made excuses. I'm teaching everything. I'd appreciate it if you'd be willing to take some of the statistics. It's not my strongest area."

Peter rose, tall and thin, like a periscope rising from a submarine. "I can't see why not. I've been hoping someone would ask. I'd be delighted. Do you think we intimidate the other faculty?"

"I don't know, but the more you can teach stats, the happier I'll be. I look forward to learning a lot from you."

He said "Pshaw," including pronouncing the P. He had a charming accent.

After that, Peter taught almost all the statistics. I usually sat in the back, learning along with the students. It was a pleasure to meet Peter's wife, Jill, and his sweet young son, Daniel, who completed my education by explaining that what I called potato chips were "crisps" and what I called French fries were "chips." Our families became good friends.

I'll never forget the day he watched me lecture about Lot Quality Assurance Surveys. This is a method for finding estimates of proportions in small sample sizes. If you don't understand this, don't worry—you'll live a long and happy life without knowing the details. Peter patiently sat in the back of the room. Finally, someone asked such a difficult question about the underlying statistics I was stumped and asked Peter for help. He strode up to the front. He whispered that he wasn't familiar with LQAS methodology.

To the class, he said, "Let's see how it works if we start from the binomial theorem." He wrote a few lines of numbers on the board, derived the LQAS formula, and produced the critical insight I had missed. It was all clear.

I knew I was in the company of a great man.

CHAPTER 27
SLEEPING SICKNESS

The only store in Kampala that sold ketchup was an Italian grocery. They ran out for several weeks, so Budsy made her own ketchup. "You're not going to believe this," she said. "One of the ingredients in ketchup is mustard seeds. I had to find some wild mustard and collect the seeds myself."

While she beavered away on cooking projects, I returned to work. One day, I was snoozing with my head in my arms on my desk when a French guy with dark brown hair and intense brown eyes knocked on my office door.

"Hello, I'm Yvan Hutin of *Médecins Sans Frontières* (MSF)."

"Nice to meet you. I'm Mark White."

"I know who you are. That's why I'm here. I have an important program in the north, and I need your help."

I yawned. "Isn't the north mainly controlled by Kony and the Lord's Resistance Army (LRA)?" Kony supplemented his troops by kidnapping children. They burst into a village and entered each hut. If there were teenagers, the LRA forced them to put a hand on the machete they used to kill the parents and younger kids. Then. They took the kids to their camp in the bush, doped them up, and continued the boys' education in cruelty. They sold the girls into slavery as prostitutes.

I shook my head at Yvan, "Our cook's brother was a truck driver up there. Kony's men caught him, tied him to the steering wheel, and poured gas over his head. Then they set him alight."

Yvan raised an eyebrow. "That happens sometimes. Did they say anything about the Ten Commandments?"

"Yes, they scattered copies of the Commandments around the truck. I guess they hadn't read the one about not killing."

He smiled crookedly. "That is an occupational hazard of our work. So far, they have left us alone, perhaps because the people like us."

I couldn't help but smile. "Glad to hear it, Yvan. I regret that many people I investigate don't like me."

"Perhaps you should join MSF."

"What do you do up there?"

"Sleeping sickness is terrible there. In many villages, most of the families have someone with it."

"Jesus."

"Have you seen people with the disease?" he asked.

"No, but I studied it. As I remember, it's caused by a trypanosome that looks like an eel with a fin on its back. Mostly, tsetse flies carry the disease among cattle and wild animals, but if a fly bites you, it might inject parasites that then home in on your brain and start to eat."

"Not exactly how they taught me in France, but close enough. My goal is to eliminate sleeping sickness from Uganda."

"Good luck. We deal mostly with preventing epidemics and doing surveys."

Yvan smiled. "Precisely. MSF needs a survey to identify where the sleeping sickness problem is worst so we can set up clinics there. Have you traveled to the north?" I'm sure he assumed I never had.

Proudly, I said, "Once to a measles epidemic. Also, Gilbert, Professor Bukenya, took me on vacation to cruise the Nile on the northern border."

"The famous Professor Bukenya. You vacation with him?"

"A few times."

He looked uncomfortable. "Do you mind if I sit down? It's tiring standing."

"Oh God, of course. Please. Our conversation is so interesting, I forgot."

He sat.

"On that trip, Gilbert showed me how to identify tsetse flies."

"Good place for it."

"We took a tour boat down the Nile. I was standing by the railing of our tour boat when Gilbert pointed to a big fly on my arm. He said, 'That's a tsetse fly.'"

"Did it bite you?" Yvan asked with clinical interest.

"No, I brushed it off.

"I collect medical insects, so I asked Gilbert how to catch one. Gilbert climbed up to the bridge and said something to the captain, who put a microphone to his lips. 'This *muzungu* wants a tsetse fly. Please bring him some.'"

A muzungu is a foreigner, usually a white one. Little kids often walk up to you and ask, "Muzungu, give me your watch," or "Muzungu, buy me a car." They had an inflated idea of our net worth.

"Soon after the captain's announcement, a dozen passengers descended on me with flies in their fingers, napkins, and handkerchiefs. Some flies were dead, others squirming and alive. All the flies buzzing around the boat turned out to be tsetses. The people said the best way to identify a tsetse is that when it lands on you, it pushes its tail up as it puts its head down to bite you."

Yvan said, "Yes. They don't suck your blood. They take

bites out of you. Ouch. And you may find you are infected with sleeping sickness."

Just talking about tsetses made the back of my neck itch. I resisted the urge to scratch it. "Yvan, there were so many flies on that boat. You couldn't live near the river without being constantly bitten."

Yvan pulled a report from his briefcase and handed it to me. "Most bites don't transfer infection, even if the flies have the parasites. Still, there are many human infections. If you look at the report, you'll see we found about fifteen hundred cases last year."

"Fifteen hundred cases is a bunch," I said, "especially considering almost everyone who gets sleeping sickness dies."

Yvan scratched the back of his neck.

I went into epidemiologist mode. "The best and cheapest way to stop new cases would be to eliminate the tsetse flies."

"Yes, we do that. Every year we hang thousands of tsetse fly traps along the rivers."

"How do the traps work?"

"Don't ask me who figured this out," he smiled, "but the flies' favorite color is bright blue. We make blue fabric cubes with a hole in the bottom. A fly is attracted to the trap. It can't resist going up the hole, where it finds itself entangled in an insecticide-soaked net. It's very effective, though you have to replace the insecticide every few months.

"Finding and treating hundreds of human cases is another matter. To be sure of the diagnosis, we must persuade people to allow us to do a lumbar puncture." This is a tall order since you must stick a hollow needle into the person's back between the vertebrae and drain a little fluid surrounding the spine. It's not painless, but it is usually more scary than painful.

Yvan offered free treatment. It was easy when people

knew what happens with sleeping sickness. You get too sleepy to eat; eventually, you waste away and die.

He said, "First, we set up clinics in villages with many cases. People were desperate to be treated.

"Gradually, we got them all treated and then sent teams to nearby villages, and so on. We've finished the highest prevalence areas and must decide where to go next. That's why I'm here, to ask you to help with the survey."

"If we want to eradicate the disease, we need to find every case, including early ones with no symptoms."

"It's not easy because we must do a lumbar puncture on everybody in the house. As you can imagine, this requires a lot of persuading if nobody's seen cases in the village or nearby. So we hope to sample as few houses as possible."

I stood and picked up my cup. Yvan stared. "Where are you going?"

"To get us some tea and, if we're lucky, to introduce you to Peter Smith. He's head of statistics for the London School of Tropical Medicine and Hygiene. I think we can help you."

Peter was in his office. It was larger than mine, so we moved there. I gave Peter a cup of tea and got Yvan settled.

As soon as we sat, Yvan told his story. I said, "Looks like a perfect case for LQAS."

Peter shook his head. "In principle, yes."

Yvan asked, "What's LQAS?"

Peter had been researching LQAS. He found a blank sheet of paper and sketched out a normal curve. "Normally, we'd collect subjects and then identify the mean of our sample. Then we use statistics to estimate how close the real population value is likely to be to our sample mean."

Yvan leaned back. His eyes squinted. "Yes, I remember that from college…" he said, his voice trailing off.

"This is inefficient if you are working with small numbers. If your population is a village of only fifty people, there won't be enough people, and it will be impossible to calculate a confidence interval or p-value for comparisons."

Peter looked up from under his white brows. "They have this problem in factories where they make products in lots of, say, ball bearings. You want to guarantee that the number of defective bearings is below a certain level. Say you want no more than one percent that don't work."

I stood up and got more tea, avoiding getting involved in the math.

Yvan sipped from his cup. "I think I see. The sick people are the defective bearings."

Peter looked up from his paper. "Exactly. Of course, we must assume that people and ball bearings aren't all that different. Since they are, we must always keep this in mind as we interpret the results."

I chimed in. "When you do LQAS, you decide where the limit is. You calculate how many people you need to sample to be reasonably sure. Say you want to find villages with at least one case of sleeping sickness. If you collect this many people and all are negative, then it is likely the village is free of sleeping sickness.

"If you find a single case, the village is a high-risk area and needs to be treated. It takes far less money and time than regular surveys."

In his excitement, Yvan had drunk all his tea. Yvan slammed the cup on the table. *"Voilà!"*

And so began our collaboration and friendship.

Yvan was a pacifist, which complicated his life during the violence of Uganda at the time, especially in the north where his project worked. He lived in a big mansion on Tank Hill, the fanciest neighborhood in the country. He fired the security guards as soon as he arrived but allowed a little guy with a bow and arrow to stay. "I instructed him not to shoot but to make a lot of noise if someone tried to get in." Incredibly, it worked, and nobody raided his house.

A few weeks after Yvan moved in, his wife and small girls flew in from Paris. They arrived at Entebbe late at night. Yvan picked them up and drove the family to Kamala. On the way up the Tank Hill, Yvan pulled a stop sign when a big man stepped out of the shadows. Yvan rolled down his window and asked, "Do you need a ride?"

"Get out of the car and leave the keys," the shadow man said. He held up what looked like a gun. When Yvan opened the door, the light revealed the bandit was holding his hand with his index finger out like a gun barrel and his thumb like a hammer.

"For Christ's sake!" Yvon said. He slammed the door, and they drove up the hill.

His wife and daughters flew back to Paris the next day. So he was alone in the big house.

Budsy and I became his Ugandan family. He'd invite us for long, boozy lunches on Saturdays. Yvan was a great cook. Once, he showed us what he described as an old French cavalry trick. He scored the neck of a wine bottle with a table knife and then tapped the bottleneck. The top broke off smoothly. I could practice on a whole case of wine and probably not get it right.

Nearly a year later, Yvan returned to my office with the survey results and the hundreds of people they'd treated.

That was the 1980s. Over the years, the incidence of human sleeping sickness continued to fall, and in 2022, WHO certified Uganda free from human sleeping sickness.

Yvan and MSF saved thousands of lives. They left a great legacy.

CHAPTER 28
IN THE LION'S DEN

As we drove between epidemics, Budsy and I saw a few zebras and warthogs in the countryside but no other big game. So we decided to go on a safari to celebrate six months in Uganda. We loaded into our reliable little Suzuki Vitara and headed for Queen Elizabeth National Park in the Rwenzori Mountains on the border with Congo, which was then named Zaire. At one point, we asked a farmer for directions. The tall man wearing overalls smiled and said, "*Mzee*, you are standing on the border. Every morning I drive my cows to eat grass in Zaire, and we return to Uganda in the evening. They are international cows."

Mzee is the Swahili term of respect used for elders. I asked people to call me Bwana, which means mister. Nobody ever did.

We soon found the park and settled into our comfortable room in the lodge, which looked like a motel made of reddish-brown bricks. A man at the desk had us fill out forms. "There are three important things I must tell you."

He waited until he was sure he had our full attention. "First, the animals that kill the most people in parks are hippos. Second, cape buffalos are the next big killers. Third, avoid getting near other animals, including elephants."

Piqued, Budsy looked up at the desk clerk. "Hippos stay in the water. How can they be dangerous?"

"Madam," the clerk said, "you must avoid getting in the water with them. The males can be territorial. They are dangerous on land, too. Hippos need to eat about ninety pounds of grass a day, so they climb out of the water in the cool night to eat grass. They try to stay close to the river to escape if lions attack. If a noise scares them, they bolt back to the water and run over anything that gets in the way—including people."

We retreated to our room for a nap before dinner at eight. Most of our friends ate much later. In my opinion, Ugandans eat unnecessarily late. The closer you are to the equator, the faster the sun sets. It is usually dark by dinner. The road we took to get to the park ran along the equator. Every so often, you find a great bronze circle along the road, indicating the equator. I imagined a thick invisible cable going through the loops. Great for photo ops.

Dinner was hearty and delicious. As we listened to the exciting reports of our fellow diners, we couldn't wait to see the animals. We went through the restaurant's double doors and were about halfway to our room when we turned a corner and nearly bumped into a giant hippo chewing on the grass and flowers. It raised its face, and we saw wiry hairs poking out over its immense gray snout. The hippo shot steamy humidity from its enormous nostrils every time it took a noisy breath.

Slowly, we backed away. Going back to the restaurant seemed pointless, so we edged away and walked about fifteen feet out into the darkness and away from the monster.

Budsy said, "Do you think there are lions around?"

I imagined a pair of sneaky lionesses stalking us but tried to put on a good face. "The hippo would know if a lion were close."

"Let's say there is a lion," Budsy persisted. "If we run, it will charge. Let's walk slowly, and maybe we can get in the door before it pounces."

We reached the flimsy door of our room and launched ourselves onto the bed. That door couldn't keep a monkey out, let alone something as big as a lion or hippo. We held each other for a long time. Our adventure had begun.

There were no hippos early the following day when we collected our box lunch and drove off along the dusty road. The guy at the desk advised us that the best times to see animals are dawn or dusk when they are most active, and there was no need to worry that other safaris had driven them away. About ten minutes later, a string of baby warthogs streamed across the road in a funny, stiff run, their little tails standing up like antennas.

I wondered how those cute little piglets could grow into vicious warthogs. Suddenly, daddy hog placed himself between us and the babies. He stood about four feet at the shoulder and sported fierce twisted, yellowing tusks. He put his head down as if bowing to us, pawed the dirt, and shook his head back and forth. A challenge! Our little Vitara wasn't all that much bigger than he was. Budsy said, "That bastard could knock the radiator out."

"If he does, we'll have enough spareribs and chops to feed the whole lodge."

She grimaced. "Not funny. Don't back up, or he'll think we're weak and charge."

Flies buzzed in and out the windows as we sat in the heat. We could smell animal dung. Finally, the monster raised its head and trotted after his babies with dignity.

In the following days, we saw a pair of elephants with their trunks twisted together. They seemed to be either fighting or falling in love. There were giraffes, buffalo, and antelopes. But no lions.

Finally, we asked the guy at the lodge desk. He pulled out a map and traced a long route across the entire park. "People aren't supposed to live here, but some have moved deep into the forest in the center. Every time a lion eats somebody, the villagers put out poisoned meat and kill it. They deny it, but I'm sure that's what they do. That's why the lions are only at the far edge.

"The best time to see them is at dawn or dusk. You don't want to be out there at night, so I recommend a very early start."

So it was that we headed out into the morning gloom. The roads got smaller and rougher. I asked Budsy to drive, and she agreed with delight.

You could see the sun peeking over the horizon when we came to a long straightaway. Budsy laughed, "Watch this!" and floored the accelerator. We spent more time in the air than on the ground as we bounced along. Ahead, we saw a giant mud puddle. Budsy laughed, "I'll take it straight on so we won't slide sideways."

About halfway into the puddle, the Vitara lurched to a stop. She hit the steering wheel, and I hit the dashboard. Horrified, we saw a line of bubbles marking our car's outline, steadily sinking into the thick reddish-brown mud. We were sinking.

Budsy said, "Shit, we can't open the doors without flooding the floor."

I launched myself out my window to solid ground, then walked around and helped her out.

Behind us, we heard a snort like a hippo. We turned and looked into the gleaming little red eyes of an immense cape buffalo. *Son of a bitch.* Instinctively, we reached for each other's hands.

The buffalo glared, whipping its tail back and forth idly. Everything smelled like the mud of the wallow, including us.

We stood like Hansel and Gretel in the fairy tale.

"I'm sorry," Budsy said.

"Don't worry. I'd probably have done the same thing. We

need a plan to get away from here and find some help." Guilt was the last thing on my mind.

"If he chases us, we can climb that candelabra tree," she said.

The tree was a twenty-foot-tall cactus. Inch-long spines poked in long lines on each leaf.

"It looks like our only choice. I doubt we could outrun the buffalo."

Budsy considered the buffalo. "We could dodge."

I pictured Budsy dodging back and forth as the buffalo bore down on me.

"Yes, and we could yell at it. Hell, we could call for help."

She smiled. "We haven't seen anybody for miles. More likely, we'd attract lions."

"We know there's nobody behind us. Our best shot is to follow the road and hope to get out of the park and find somebody," she said faintly.

"Good point," I said and led us in a circle about fifteen yards from the buffalo. It ignored us.

We padded down the road. The sun was well up now, so the lion menace was reduced—we hoped. We constantly scanned the park around us. Breezes ruffled the grass. Blessedly, there were no large animals or poisonous snakes. A half hour or so later, we heard faint singing and voices. We weren't as quiet as we thought because a mob of little kids ran toward us. Our entourage led us to the village—some huts and a central enclosure.

They only knew two words of English: "beer" and "shillings." We knew they understood our dilemma because they laughed and slapped each other's backs. We made a little charade of driving into the waterhole. The leader mimicked pushing the car and then made a big circle with his arms. "Beer." He wanted a case of beer. And they say love is the international language.

The chief signaled the young men, and we set off to get

the car. The entire village followed. Nursing mothers, old people, and of course, the kids. In their excitement, some of them orbited us like impatient dogs. When we got to the buffalo, a kid picked up a little stone and threw it at its face. The giant animal backed up and then turned and loped away. It was the first thing the villagers taught us.

The car was something else. We were relieved to see it hadn't sunk deeper, so the mud was still below the windows. Everyone crowded around the wallow. This was more than they'd bargained for. Nobody moved at first. Then a big man took my hand and stepped into the mud. He pointed to my watch, an antique Rolex my grandfather had given me. I shook my head no. Another man pointed to Budsy's sun hat. She firmly held it down with her hand.

The chief and I reopened negotiations. He asked for two cases. I agreed.

The young men stepped into the wallow and put their hands on the car. The chief shouted for them to stop. He led Budsy to the car and helped her into the driver's seat. Then an old man began to chant in a slow rhythm.

Nothing happened. They tried again and again. No joy. Finally, the whole tribe waded in, including women, teenagers, and old men. With a tremendous flatulent sucking burp, the wallow gave up the car. Budsy turned the key. Amazingly, it started. Between the villagers and Budsy, the car rolled out onto the road.

The muddy villagers sang a victory song. We all shared muddy embraces and a few kisses. I kept enough money for gas and gave all the rest to the chief.

I drove slowly back, and we arrived at the lodge at about 1:00 p.m. There were muddy handprints all over the white paint. We sat alone at a small table and hoped for a quiet dinner.

Our fellow diners asked what had happened to our car.

Budsy smiled. "What? Somebody put handprints on our car?"

I said, "We'll complain to the manager first thing in the morning."

I am profoundly grateful we never saw a lion.

CHAPTER 29
THIRSTY WORK

A few weeks after the lion safari, trouble struck closer to home.

When Ugandans talk about someone from their native village, they call them brother or sister. This led Budsy and me to some serious misunderstandings at first. Our landlady recommended her "sister" Marie to work as our maid, and she brought a friend named Carolyn, who cooked for us. Marie was a happy, big-hearted young lady, maybe eighteen years old. Carolyn was older, smaller, and less talkative. Things worked well for a while, but one day Gerald, the alcoholic house boy (a "brother" of our landlord), brought me a letter he had found in Carolyn's room. Marie held out the letter. "It's from Boxer."

She wrung her hands as if washing them. "Boxer lives two houses down the street. He is the leader of our Olympic Boxing Team. He and Carolyn are friends." She looked down. "I think they are lovers."

She read, "Dearest Darling, You know I love you, and I want us to go away together as soon as I earn enough money. But not this way.

"You are so small and sweet when we are alone. I cannot believe you want to kill the muzungus and take their things. I know they are rich, but the police and army would certainly catch us if we kidnapped them. These are evil ideas. Let us forget them.

"Be patient, my sweet girl, and soon I will earn enough money to make you my wife, and we will have a bigger house than the muzungus, and you will have your own cook and maid.

"I love you always, my dearest darling, Boxer."

It froze the blood in our hearts. Outside, our cat pounced on a rat, and they scuffled briefly until he killed it.

I heard breathing behind me. I could feel it on the back of my neck. I lurched forward into Gerald and spun to see Budsy, eyes aflame.

"I heard everything from the hall. We've got to get that bitch before she gets us," Budsy exploded. "If we have to kill her before she kills us, it's fine with me."

Budsy had proposed killing someone before. She was born in the Batangas Province of the Philippines to a matriarchal tribe where women carry large knives called *balisongs* and are reputed to be witches. She had a blazing temper and an extensive vocabulary to express it. She is the only person I've seen get hopping mad. It was a fearsome sight. When a young man impregnated her niece, she learned he wanted to join the police force. She bribed the officers who were interviewing him to kill him. She only told me about this when she learned they only beat him up. Lucky thing. He later married the niece.

"Buds, let's not go overboard."

She grabbed my shoulders and shook me. "Do you want to wait until she and her boyfriend come through that door with fucking axes and leave us hacked to pieces, drowned in our own blood?"

Budsy was only about four feet eight inches tall, but she seemed to tower above us in her wrath. She turned on Maria. "Where is she? Bring her here right now."

"I'm sorry, mum. She's gone."

The next day, I consulted Gilbert and showed him the letter.

"What are you going to do with this, White?" Gilbert said gravely.

"That's why I'm here."

"Well, your choices are to beat her, discharge her, or take her to the police."

I said, "This is the sort of thing I would take to the police in the US."

"Well, that's appropriate here, too," Gilbert said gravely.

He seemed oddly disengaged, not telling me something important. Only his eyes moved as I stood and left the room.

I drove home, where Budsy and Marie told me that Caroline had taken her clothes and left to stay with her brother, who was working at a house nearby. Marie and Gerald persuaded the bother to give Carolyn up. She came back spitting and cursing. It was easy to see her as someone who would've killed us in cold blood. We loaded her into the car and drove her to the police station, a big round tin hut with a thatched roof. Six or seven policemen busied themselves with various tasks in the sunshine.

A man who looked to be the chief met me, and I explained things. He pulled Carolyn out of the car and called two policemen, who took Carolyn into the darkness of the hut. To our horror, they took Marie as well. Then the chief sat me down by a desk, and we began filling out a five-page form that listed details about our complaint. We were about a page in when I heard the first scream from inside the hut when I looked up. The police chief smiled at me and said, "Justice begins."

I looked around and saw the police had opened all the windows. The chief said, "I want people to hear the screams —an example for the children." A crowd of women held small children up to the windows to enjoy the spectacle.

A couple of questions later, I could hear both women screaming and begging. It was too much. Looking in the door, I saw both young women had lost control of their bladders and bowels. A policeman holding a rubber cable forced them to clean it up. Then he began beating them again. He didn't seem to be asking any questions.

I bolted from my chair. "Stop! I withdraw the charges."

The policeman smiled slowly. "Sir, once I begin this form, the inquiry is official. It's not in your hands anymore. The sooner you finish, the sooner you can go home."

"I've heard that women get raped in the prisons."

"Yes, they do. You can think of it as part of the punishment."

"But she hasn't been judged guilty yet. A lot of people have AIDS here. Isn't she likely to get it?"

"That is true. It is an unfortunate part of the present historical situation we find ourselves in."

I stared at the articulate monster before me. His eyes narrowed on me, and a small smile danced on his lips. He seemed to be waiting. I got the idea.

"I know how hard you work, sir, and I can see I've caused you a great deal of trouble. Is there anything I can do to repay you?"

"Well, it's thirsty work interrogating people in this heat. I suppose a case of beer would make things easier for all of us and let things cool down."

"I'll be right back."

I was back in fifteen minutes with a case of Nile Specials, Uganda's most delicious and famous beer. It came in huge bottles, at least twice as big as regular beer bottles. The policeman got up from his chair and smiled appreciatively. Another led the two girls, surprisingly little bruised, out to my car.

Carolyn didn't speak. As we arrived home, Budsy shouted, "Get out." Carolyn went to her room, came out with a large cloth bundle, and hurried out the front door. We never saw her again. Unfortunately, this didn't mean we didn't hear her. Every Sunday, she called us and said things like, "I'm sure I'll see you this week. I'm looking forward to visiting your home. We have so much to catch up on."

At first, Carolyn's calls were annoying, but over the months, we became concerned she might do something. I decided to see the neighborhood Resistance Chairman. He was like the mayor of the neighborhood. He was a tough guy. Once Budsy called me at work to tell me that his bodyguards had shot two men down in the street and that the bodies still lay there hours later. I came home from work and talked to the chairman.

"They came to rob me and kill me. What else could I do?"

"I take your point. But the bodies in the street are a public health problem. Let me send a vehicle from Mulago Hospital to pick them up."

"I want to leave them in the street a little longer to deter others from making the same mistake," he said. "Please sit down. I'll order us some tea."

I wanted to spend as little time as possible with this man, so I got to the point and told him the story of Carolyn's plot to murder us and her threatening phone calls.

There was nothing to do but accept his offer of tea, and we sat in his living room. "So you see that your revolutionary taxes are well spent. It is unfortunate, very unfortunate, that you didn't come to me sooner."

"Why?"

"Because she was working for an army officer about a half mile from here. Last week she ran away, and he found she had taken all his money and checkbook. Did she steal money from you?"

"Some."

"Well, you have something to be thankful for." He rose, and I walked with him to the door. "I want my constituents to know that I'm serving. Please share the story of how my men killed the two bandits. I've put Carolyn's name and picture on the government network and hope somebody will catch her soon and send her to jail."

This time, I thought of her in jail with grim pleasure. "I look forward to it, sir."

CHAPTER 30
THE WARAGI CURE

Budsy remained healthy after the murder plot—except once when she got a nasty cold. She lay coughing on the couch in my office. "This God damned cough is going to kill me," she gasped. "It's been over a week. I used up the last of the cough syrup yesterday."

Just then, Wamuyu Maina walked in. A good-looking woman, Wamuyu was a refugee from Kenya. She was from a Kikuyu family that farmed in the countryside. The famously photogenic Maasai herders burned them out to provide more grazing land. She ended up in Uganda, studying with us.

"Budsy, do you know what we take for bad coughs?" Wamuyu asked.

Budsy coughed. "No, but I'll try anything."

"Are you bringing anything up?"

Wamuyu smiled. "The country people make a forest gin called *waragi*. When I had a cough, my mother would give me a tablespoon of waragi and a little honey."

Budsy coughed. "Did it help?"

"I honestly can't remember. I'm here, though, so maybe it did."

Budsy lurched out of the room to find John, the driver, to

buy some waragi. John said, "I'll have the waragi for you in two hours."

Budsy screeched, "There must be a way to get it sooner! This cough is killing me."

"I'll hurry, ma'am. Please give me ten thousand shillings for the bottle."

Budsy handed him the money—about ten dollars—and squeezed his hand so hard he winced.

An hour later, John delivered the waragi and five thousand shillings in change. We headed home. After a quick dinner, Budsy poured the waragi into a pan and added a few tablespoons of honey. "I think it'll be safest to boil it," she said, and boil it she did.

She tasted a tablespoon full and made a face. "Doesn't taste half-bad. Kind of like regular gin." Ten minutes later, she had a coughing fit. "This warm honey soothes my throat," she croaked. She poured herself a half cup and sipped.

I graded papers for an hour or so. Then I went to check on Budsy. She was slumped back into the chair, her face red and her eyes glowing. "I don't usually like to drink, but this stuff hits the spot. Can't beat the price, either."

She was toasted, a little drunk. I took the waragi away. She didn't notice.

Around midnight she asked me to help her to bed, where she wordlessly lay down, fully clothed, and began snoring. At least she wasn't coughing.

I feared she might have a hangover in the morning, but she didn't complain. "I'm just tired, she said. She managed to shower and put on clean clothes. I gave her a cup of coffee. She sipped it, then nibbled a corner of a slice of toast and marmalade. No coughing.

Budsy slept away most of the day in my office. Eventually, she woke, took a Kleenex from her purse, and blew her nose. "I haven't coughed since yesterday."

She wiped her eyes. "I think this stuff is like chemo-therapy for cold viruses."

"How's waragi like chemotherapy? You think it might cure your metastases?" I asked.

"It either kills the cough, or it kills you. I would have been happy with either."

Despite her miraculous cure, I was nervous about her. She'd grown weaker in the last year. Knowing she'd need specialized care, I looked for a job in the US. Steve Thacker, the head of my center, the Epidemiology Program Office, announced he was replacing the director of the global training programs. I applied.

The night before my interview, I had dinner with consul-tants from other programs in Hungary, Zimbabwe, and Italy.

The guy from Zimbabwe was bitter. "We all know Steve will appoint a woman. I think it's because he has two daugh-ters. He actually says he's a feminist. It's so unfair."

Nancy Binkin, the consultant from Italy, said, "Don't you think it's unfair that most of CDC top management is men? So's middle management."

"There are more quality men in the pool." Zimbabwe smiled thinly.

Mary Agocs from Hungary glared. "If you must know, Steve already offered it to me, and I refused."

Zimbabwe ordered another round of beers and buried his nose in his mug.

Refreshed, I swallowed and burped. "There's no need to fight. Every director has been an American with no international experience and no training experience. Top management just appoints whoever sucks up. Maybe Steve owes somebody a favor."

"I don't believe that," Nancy said. "Steve's the most ethical person at CDC. He'd never do that."

We left the bar one at a time, deep in our thoughts.

The following day I arrived late for my appointment with

Steve. Knowing I had no chance, I dressed in a T-shirt and jeans. I took the chair he offered and put my feet up on the table in front of me.

"I want you to tell me honestly, Mark, what you think of the program."

Having nothing to lose, I told him the truth. "Steve, most of the Atlanta staff haven't taught, so their advice isn't much help. The field staff is at the bottom of the totem pole, so we have to put up with Atlanta staff inviting themselves to our countries to 'help.' Of course, they charge their expenses to our budgets."

I stood and turned to go. "I want to thank you for the opportunity to let you know how it looks from the field.

"Don't you want to know if you got the job?"

I took my hand off the doorknob and faced him.

"I want you to do the job." He smiled.

"After all the negative stuff I told you?"

"Because of what you told me. My observations are the same as yours. I trust your judgment. The other consultants thought you'd be good as well."

Unfortunately for Steve, I had just read a book on negotiating. "There's just one thing, Steve. I left CDC, and now I'm coming back."

"No worries, I'll give you the same level position you had when you left."

I sat back down in the chair. "Here's the thing. I have had a lot of experience in the six years since I left. I need to get credit for those years."

"I can probably arrange that."

"Also, Steve, Budsy's breast cancer recurred, and she's got lung metastases. And I've got two kids in college. I think it would be most fair if you pay me what Rockefeller paid to help with these extraordinary expenses. I think that's reasonable."

"How much did Seth pay you?"

"Three hundred thousand dollars."

He stood, knocking his chair back. Steve was a tall, muscular man, an athlete who played basketball at lunch. He could be intimidating.

"That included my housing, security, and travel," I admitted. "But I'm hoping to give you the range."

His face reddened. "I don't have to give you the job."

"I know, Steve. I appreciate your faith in me. If I had a choice, this would be my dream job. But I need to care for my family. My next choice is to go back to doing clinical infectious diseases in New York City. I'll miss epidemiology, but the private sector pays enough for me to care for Budsy and the kids."

He shook his head. "I'll offer the absolute most I can. It'll be a lot less than you want. Even so, this is gonna cost me, White."

"Thank you, Steve. I swear I'll produce so much you'll get your money's worth."

"I doubt it. Close the door behind you."

I waited until I was through the door before I smiled.

For the next two months, I didn't hear from Steve. Then an irritable administrator called to finalize the details of hiring me. "I'm afraid Steve violated the regs when he offered you so much money. The best I can do is to reinstate your old rank."

"Tell Steve goodbye for me." I hung up.

That night, Budsy looked across the bed at me. "You're usually such a lousy bargainer. I'm proud you hung tough." Her dark brown eyes teared up, and she snuggled up, put her arms around me, and hugged hard. "I don't know what we'll do, Mark. Thank you for protecting me."

"Don't worry, Buds, I'll call around for Infectious Diseases jobs."

"Let's hope you get an offer. Don't be such a hard-ass next time."

I kissed her eyelids. "I'll be grateful for whatever I find."

As it turned out, Steve's associate director for management, a wonderful grandmotherly woman named Barbara Holloway, called a couple of weeks later. "I'm so disappointed you got that stupid call. I'm handling your case now."

"Thanks, Barb. I despaired."

"Oh God, don't be so dramatic. I want you to know that Steve had to go all the way to CDC executive committee and convince them you are a distinguished scientist so he can pay you more."

"What?"

"With your record, it was a tough sell. He had to trade some big favors. You will take what I offer, and I don't want to hear from you until you arrive ready to work."

"Yes, thanks. I'm in your hands. Fax me the paperwork, and I'll sign it. Goodbye."

"Don't you want to know about your salary and benefits?"

"I trust you and Steve. Tell him thanks and that I'm proud to be on his team."

"Good call, Mark. Say hi to Budsy."

CHAPTER 31
A SHOCKING DEVELOPMENT

efore my Rockefeller contract ended, I found a replacement for myself, Larry Marum, who'd been doing AIDS epidemiology in Kampala. Budsy arranged our move, and some guys appeared at the house and boxed most of our stuff up. It all seemed to be coming together. We were leaving in two days.

I got up early to finalize grades for the last papers. It must have been around 6:00 a.m. I put on some underwear and padded barefoot down the hall to our office. I reached out and turned on the desk lamp. The world turned to black-and-white dots. Everything vibrated. There was no time or space. I felt myself falling back into blackness. Later, the room came back into focus. The lamp lay on the floor a foot away from me. When I tried to talk, I made a hoarse bark.

Son of a bitch.

My left thumb, the one I'd touched the lamp with, hurt like hell. I saw a white blister forming.

I managed to stagger out to the bedroom and wake Budsy.

"Buds, I was electrocuted."

"Thank God you're OK."

"I'm not. My left shoulder hurts." I raised my arm and felt a claw of pain ripping into my shoulder joint.

Budsy stared at my shoulder. "No swelling or bruising yet. I'll make you a sling."

"Thanks. I saw a guy who repaired optical disk drives who got a big shock in his arm. He said he wanted to see what happens."

"What happens?"

"The electricity made the muscles jerk so hard they pulled his humerus out of the shoulder joint. An orthopedic surgeon popped it back in. If that's what it is, I'll be in a lot of pain for a few seconds, but I'll be better in a few minutes."

Fortunately for me, Larry Marum, my replacement, worked part-time as the embassy doctor. I called him up. "Larry, I've been electrocuted. Could you prescribe codeine pills? My shoulder hurts like a bear."

Larry slowed his voice the way you do when talking to a lunatic. "Sure, but I think I should see you first. Meet me at the clinic."

"It's six a.m. I don't want to drag you in."

"It's no bother," he said carefully. "Besides, it's ten to seven now."

Larry, a thin, brown-haired guy with a goatee, said, "First, I think we should get an EKG."

"You don't think the shock might have damaged my heart?"

"Probably not, but I'd like to document things. You might have a new arrhythmia."

He and Budsy strapped the leads on me, and he ran the test, including a long strip to check that my rhythm was OK. It was. Then he checked for nerve damage by touching my fingers and checking my bicipital reflex. Finally, he reached up my arm and gently pressed his fingers into the shoulder joint to feel for a dislocation.

I screamed.

Larry said, "I think we'll need an X-ray before we go

further." The clinic was too small to justify an X-ray technician or machine, so he gave me the address of a clinic in Kampala.

Budsy drove carefully, but still, I shrieked when my shoulder hit the seat wrong.

"Try not to embarrass yourself. You sound like a baby."

"Thanks, Florence Nightingale."

I knew things were serious after the Ugandan radiologist looked at my X-ray and immediately took a second one. This usually means the radiologist is making a copy for his collection of images of horrible diseases.

He stuck my film on a light board. The upper third of my humerus was gone, replaced by tiny sharp shards and what looked like sand.

Budsy leaned forward to study the image. "No wonder you cried so much."

"Buds, this really, really hurts. I need some codeine."

We drove back to the clinic and showed the film to Larry. His first thought was, "You should have gotten me a copy."

"Sorry. Can you prescribe me something for this pain? It's getting worse by the minute."

"I don't know. I've never had to write for narcotics here."

Budsy stood up. "My oncologist prescribed fentanyl patches in case I get pain from metastases. I'll slap a couple of patches on you, and you should be fine."

It turned out I felt more than fine; I felt great. I corrected the papers, then Budsy drove me to the office. Soon my fellow doctors brought their friends to see my famous X-ray. The head of the orthopedic department at Mulago looked at the film confidently. "The best thing to do would be to disarticulate it and take the arm off."

"Woah," I said. "I emailed my doctor in the States, and he says they have a prosthesis."

"Great." the orthopedist said. "Have them FedEx a couple

of different sizes, and I'll put one in. Can't be more difficult than doing a hip."

Budsy gently put a hand on his chest. "No thanks. I've already called British Airways, and we have tickets for tomorrow's flight."

"Good luck," the surgeon said. "I look forward to seeing how it works out."

We drove home and found the packers finishing up. Budsy put Sunshine, her nasty yellow tabby tomcat, into his travel box. She'd called the airline, and they told her to drop him off at baggage six hours before the flight in his carrier box, which she did.

Budsy had made First Class reservations, so we whizzed through the line. We sat in the big seats, and Budsy had just finished fastening my seatbelt when a big man in a black, double-breasted suit with a pearl-gray tie appeared in the aisle.

"I'm in charge of baggage for this fight," he said.

"Thank God," Budsy said. "Take good care of my cat."

"Unfortunately, madam, the cat wasn't brought to the baggage office in time, so I won't be able to allow him on the plane."

Budsy stepped into the aisle. The guy wanted a bribe, but we were too upset to realize it.

"My cat comes on this flight."

"No, and I advise you to calm down," he pushed his index finger into the center of her chest.

She grabbed the finger and bent it back. The manager yipped in pain. She kept bending, and he knelt to keep her from breaking his finger. Tears streamed from his eyes. Traditionally women in Uganda must kneel to speak to a man. Budsy's move must have humiliated the manager.

"My cat comes on this flight or by God . . ."

"Yes, madam. Let me go, and I promise your cat will be on the flight."

Budsy sat down and sipped her Coke as the baggage manager scuttled toward the exit.

Sunshine had as nice a trip as someone in the baggage hold can be expected to have.

My sister, Marty Jo, had convinced an orthopedic surgeon from their church that I was a "medical missionary," which was partly true. He operated for free. I later brought him a selection of African masks.

I started my new job at CDC a few weeks late, but it all worked out.

After I left Uganda, one of my graduates, Freddie Ssengooba, a fine economist, got hold of my lamp and fixed the short. It still has pride of place in his living room.

A couple of years later, I learned my former students faced an Ebola fever epidemic. With the African strain, the death rate can be above 50 percent. The disease spreads by contact with infected blood or secretions. It should be straightforward to stop transmission by isolating patients by wearing gloves, gowns, and masks. Unfortunately, family members often treated patients with home remedies until everybody in the house was infected. The disease spreads through ignorance, wishful thinking, and lies by politicians.

One of our graduates, Matthew Lukwya, took charge of the hospital where the patients were quarantined. He got the disease and died—the last death in the outbreak. Another graduate, Margaret Lumunu, a bright, petite veterinarian, took charge of keeping the Ebola from spreading in the community. Margaret spent weeks driving and hiking villages, convincing people to take their sick relatives to the quarantine center. She was from the Acholi tribe in the north, so she understood how people thought. She was more credible to people than a *muzungu*. In Ebola epidemics, there are always rumors that *muzungus* are trying to kill Africans to take their land.

She completed a careful survey showing exactly how the disease spread in Northern Uganda. The WHO also noticed Margaret's talents. They hired her. She became one of the leading Ebola epidemiologists in Geneva and the world.

They say the evil men do lives after them. If we're lucky, the good does, too.

Margaret was part of the good.

CHAPTER 32

MRS. CHIPPY'S LAST EXPEDITION

After my shoulder surgery, we arrived in Atlanta feeling tired and banged up. Budsy's back ached from the uneven weight of her breasts, and my shoulder was in constant pain. We both found relief when we bought a house with a Jacuzzi and settled in.

My job went well, and I soon found donors to fund new FETPs around the world, including China and a Central American region. Then, in 1999, I had to go to Vietnam to teach a course. I'd been in the country for only two days when my host called me out of the class I was teaching. "Your wife just called. She's crying. She says you need to come home right away. She has a terrible cough. She thinks she might have pneumonia."

I called Budsy and told her to go to the ER. She picked up on the first ring. "I was just a little hysterical. Sorry to scare you," she said in a high voice. She gasped, then coughed. "But come home soon. If I get sicker, I'll need you."

I left three hours later, but no direct flights were available, so it took a day and a half before I landed in Atlanta and stepped out of the taxi. Our front door was unlocked. Budsy lay on the couch, breathing quietly. Bright red blood streaked the Kleenex in her hand.

"Buds, I'm going to put you in the car, and we're going to Emory ER."

She slowly walked carefully across the room to pick up a little suitcase. "I thought so," she said in a low voice.

I took the Kleenex from her hand, wiped her lips, and kissed her forehead. I put my arms around her, and we held each other for a long time.

When the ER triage nurse looked at Budsy, she called the ICU team to come straight down. They hung several IV bags and took her upstairs. The ER nurses sat me down with a thick handful of paperwork. I agreed to pay for everything and rushed upstairs. The ICU was laid out like a flower, with little rooms around the edge like petals. Each faced in toward the nursing station. Budsy lay in one of the petals. The nurses had cranked up so she could breathe. She panted and stared at me. Her worried eyes and ballooning cheeks broke my heart.

A clerk bustled in with more forms for me to fill out and sign. I reached for my wallet to get a business card for the clerk. My pocket was empty. I'd left it at home.

Budsy coughed and wheezed. "You'll need money to get out of the pay parking lot. Take twenty dollars from my bag." She was thoughtful, even in mortal danger, and I was supposed to be taking care of her.

The ICU doctor introduced himself. He looked at her sputum, stained it for bacteria, and thought it might be bacterial pneumonia.

He told both Budsy and me this together. "Mrs. White, we'll start you on very powerful antibiotics, but it'll take them a day or so to work. Your breathing isn't efficient enough to provide oxygen to your heart and brain. I'm going to have to intubate you."

She shook her head. She was terrified now. So was I. If she needed a tube to breathe, she was in great danger. It was dawning on us now, deep in our hearts, that she might die, maybe tonight.

The ICU doc was out getting the intubation kit. I had to ask the question. "Budsy, if your heart stops, do you want us to resuscitate you?" I put my arm around her and held her firmly.

She stared me straight in the eyes. "The whole nine yards," she said. "The whole nine yards."

I could only sleep that night by taking some of the Ambien I took for jet lag. In the following weeks, I took a lot of Ambien and drank a lot of bourbon.

The ICU had no visiting hours, so relatives could stay there all day and all night if they wanted. Budsy lay in her bed, knocked out, with the endotracheal tube jutting from her mouth, connecting her to the respirator. It took regular, deep breaths.

Something was wrong with her hand. "Nurse," I asked, "why is her finger taped up?"

"She wouldn't let us take off her wedding ring, so we taped it with lots of layers to make sure nobody is tempted to steal it." I wasn't surprised she held on to her ring. Being married was important to her. She carried a copy of our marriage license in her wallet.

I brought one of her favorite books, *Mrs. Chippy's Last Expedition*, about a ship's cat with Shackleton's disastrous Antarctic expedition. Even though the crew was starving, they didn't eat Mrs. Chippy—or so they said. I spent the day reading to her. And the next day. Then it was *The Princess Bride*, then *Pride and Prejudice*. Day and night came and went as I shuttled in and out of the hospital. Budsy lay on her back, eyes bandaged to keep them from drying out. She faced the ceiling beneath a neatly folded sheet and blanket. As the days passed, her skin took on a pale, ashy hue. She seemed a bit worse every day.

Every time I came in, I put my fingers between hers,

hoping for a squeeze, but it never came. I hope she was unconscious for the whole nightmare. My breathing fell into the rhythm of the respirator. I began to feel we belonged in the half-world of the ICU.

One night I came in and found somebody had pulled the curtains of Budsy's petal tight. Maybe they were bathing her, or perhaps something bad was happening. The ICU doctor and the head nurse looked at her EKG monitor, tracing slow, regular waves. I stared. After a minute, the nurse said, "Shall we disconnect her?"

"She wants to be coded."

"We're already doing everything we'd do in a code. Your wife's tubed. Pressers are running wide open into her veins, and we have her on one hundred percent oxygen."

"Could you at least shock her?"

"Look at her EKG."

I couldn't see the usual jerky QRST waves but rather a line of long, smooth curves.

The nurse traced the EKG screen with her finger. "Look at her r wave. It's really wide."

I stared.

"You know what that means, right?"

"It means her heart muscle is dying."

The nurse nodded her head. "Yes."

Budsy lay still as the machine raised and lowered her chest. I touched her cheek and quickly kissed her cold, damp forehead—no response. For all practical purposes, she was dead already.

I looked up. "OK. Take her off the machines." I felt like I was betraying her, but there was nothing more to do.

The nurse untaped Budsy's ring and handed it to me. I slid it onto my little finger.

I didn't cry. I walked to the nursing station and asked the clerk for an autopsy permission form. I asked for a complete autopsy. I wrote a detailed description of her clinical picture.

In particular, I wanted to know whether the cancer had recurred. Also, I wanted to know what caused her pneumonia. I also owed a full report to her oncologist. Then I signed the autopsy request and walked out of the building. I felt like they'd amputated one of my arms.

As I guided the car through the darkness, I worried I might be afraid to be alone in the house. If anybody could come back from the dead and haunt me, it would be Budsy. I parked and opened the front door. My heart filled with the certainty that Budsy's ghost, or some part of her, waited in the darkness. If she was, I was sure she'd let me know by pushing a bookshelf over on me.

I closed the door behind me and stood in absolute darkness. There was no sound. I realized I'd gone from being afraid she might haunt me to hoping she would. At least I'd have something of her.

She never pushed anything over on me. Later I went to her shell collection. She'd collected most of them from her favorite snorkeling site in Anilao Bay in her native province of Batangas. The most beautiful were big cone-shaped snail shells with patterns like textile cloth. The creatures creep up on sleeping fish, flick out their long, poisonous tongues, and paralyze them. They then eat the fish. We used to joke that she was related to the cone shells because of her sharp tongue.

I carry one of her shells in a pocket of my backpack.

I always will.

CHAPTER 33

IT TAKES A YEAR

The next day, I woke in the bed Budsy and I had shared, padded into her kitchen, and made a cup of coffee. As it brewed, I wandered back to the bedroom and found her closet was open. Every dress, blouse, or pair of slacks reminded me of a time when she wore each one. I reached down, picked some culottes up off the floor, and hung them on a hanger. In the kitchen, I sat in her chair and pictured her reading about Lady Diana and drinking tea.

My sister and brother flew down from Michigan, and we went together to the crematorium. It was run by a kind Unitarian with degrees in social work and funeral directing. When I called, I hadn't asked him about money, but he charged only $300.

"I have dedicated my life to relieving the pain of grieving," he said. "We save money by using the boxes that coffins come in.

"Of course, you can buy a coffin, and the price is reasonable. I'm proud of this one. I designed it for teenagers. It was white, and friends could write goodbye messages before closing it. I won an award for it."

My businessman brother asked, "Is it patented?"

The funeral director smiled. "Of course not."

Marty Jo and Thomas stayed to help with Budsy's clothes before they flew back to Michigan.

Although Budsy was a lapsed Catholic, Scott McNabb, one of my branch chiefs, convinced a Catholic chaplain at Emory University to hold a service. The father was a bit cranky and warned us that nobody should speak for a long time during the service. He'd obviously never dealt with people from CDC. Everybody, including me, spoke for three minutes or less. Budsy's brother, Peter, had brought a dozen Filipinos I didn't know. I was fine until the service ended. Then I stood before these strangers and wept.

A couple of days later, my friend Doug Klauke's wife was cashing a check in the US Embassy in Kenya when a terrorist bomb blew her to pieces. When I attended her memorial service, a woman walked up to me and asked how well I knew her. Then she stepped back, put her hand over her mouth, and said, "You poor man."

Ouch.

I flew with Budsy's ashes to Michigan for a family memorial service and then on to the Philippines. Conky Quizon and Conchy Roces arranged a service at Anilao Bay, where Budsy loved to snorkel and explore the reef. As we climbed onto the little outrigger to sail out and distribute her ashes, I noticed several people pull plastic baggies from their pockets. To my horror, I realized they planned to keep some of Budsy's ashes. It seemed ghoulish and creepy at the time. Not anymore.

I announced that all the ashes should go into the water, not into pockets. At the center of the bay, I brought out the box of ashes and passed it around. Suddenly the wind gusted, and the ashes blew back onto our faces, like in *The Big Lebowski*. Maybe her ghost was playing tricks on us. I hope so. When I tried to brush the ashes off, I felt them disappear into my pores. Maybe some are still there.

Later I sat with Conky in her beach house. I found relief in listening to the wind whispering through the bamboo. I asked her how to say it in Tagalog: *wiswis kawayan.* Lovely words.

Back in Atlanta, I told Steve Thacker that I planned to take an extended vacation and travel around Asia to grieve.

"Don't put in for leave. Just tell us where you want to go, and we'll cut travel orders. Do some work while you're there if you can. It'll make it easier for me to sleep at night."

I drifted across the Pacific to Japan, the Philippines, then back to Vietnam to finish my teaching. My friends in Hanoi took me to a unique restaurant. As we walked toward the building, they steered me toward a big bamboo cage, the kind of thing Rambo was always escaping from. Inside was a tangle of hissing cobras.

"Mark, cobras are the bravest animals. When you eat them, it makes you brave. It will help with your pain."

"Thanks, but I'm doing OK."

A man in shorts and a white shirt pulled the door to the cage open and stirred the snakes with a hooked stick. The snakes hissed and struck at the stick.

"He wants you to choose the bravest one," a friend said.

The snake keeper looped a snake around his stick.

I said, "That one, the one on the stick."

He pulled the snake out of the cage and jabbed it toward me. I leaned back as if I were doing the limbo.

A friend said, "He says that isn't the bravest one. He'll get you a bigger one." General hilarity ensued.

Finally, the snake man hooked a giant, menacing cobra on his stick. He shook the hook and wrapped the snake around it. He smiled in pleasure. Suddenly, he pulled it out of the cage and grabbed the snake behind the head. An assistant held the tail. The assistant stretched the snake and arched it so its belly pointed toward me. The snake man pulled a cloth out of a brandy snifter, washed the snake's belly, and slit it down the middle with a razor. I swear I heard a zipping noise. Then he cut out the heart, studied it, smiled, and dropped it into a snifter. Then he felt around and pulled out what must have been the gall bladder and squirted some into the snifter. Then he cut off the snake's head, filled the snifter with blood, and topped it with brandy.

Gravely, he handed me the snifter. My friend whispered in my ear. "This is a great honor. You must drink it now while the heart is still beating. Swallow it all down. Don't chew."

I put my head back and slid the warm, unholy mixture down my stunned throat. I swear I could feel my heart beating in my chest and the snake's heart beating in my stomach for the rest of the evening.

The house specialty was snake fifteen ways, and we spent the evening trying each one. Snake soup is good, but the spareribs aren't worth the trouble. As the evening wore down, I felt pleased that I survived the trial without shaming myself.

Then my host rose. "Mark, what's the bravest part of the snake?"

I knew this one. "The heart." I pointed to my belly, and everyone laughed.

"No! The testes. So we must finish with testicular wine!" Everyone at our table applauded, and soon, the whole restaurant was cheering and laughing as a waiter took a large glass jar of what looked like an anatomical specimen in formalin. The specimen was the long fleshy testicle of a snake. Thank God we only sipped the wine.

I flew back via Lyon in Southern France. I'd been to several WHO meetings there. It's a small city ringed by rivers. Like Boston, it's big enough for interesting historical and cultural things and small enough to get to know well. The people are warm, even if you don't speak French. They say it has the best food in France, but on that trip, I went to the little grocery near my hotel and got bread, butter, jam, and ice cream. I wanted to be alone.

I felt better when I got back home to Atlanta. Marty Jo had

told me that grief takes you every day for about a year. After that, it visits less often. Of course, it never goes away. That's fine with me.

Budsy's wedding ring fit perfectly on my left little finger. I gave her engagement ring to her niece. A few months later, I dropped the wedding ring into the grass in Luneta Park, which was full of people begging or sleeping in the bushes. I hope it did a lot of good for whoever picked it up. Budsy would like that, I think.

When I returned to Atlanta, I called Emory University Hospital several times for the autopsy results. They wouldn't release the report to me until I pointed out that, legally, the information belonged to me. Finally, the ICU doctor called me and said she had disseminated *Aspergillus niger*, an overwhelming fungal infection. There was no sign of cancer. I sent the report to my brother-in-law, the oncologist who generously gave her experimental treatment.

Aspergillus niger is, I think, the main ingredient in soy sauce. Budsy used to buy it in five-gallon cans. I guess the aspergillus finally settled the score. For a long time, I refused to eat soy sauce.

I later reconsidered, and now I eat it as often as possible.

Take that, black fungus.

CHAPTER 34
MEETING GÉRARD

About six months after Budsy died, I went to a meeting in France to help organize a new nongovernmental organization of epidemiology training programs. I flew into Geneva and took a bus into the mountains to Annecy.

Wet snow slanted onto my back and hair as I faced the great wooden doors to Dr. Charles Mérieux's twelfth-century abbey. There seemed to be only a few lights on deep inside the building. I pounded on the thick doors, shivering because I only had a suit coat. In the dark behind me, my taxi slid down the driveway and disappeared down the slushy mountain road.

I hadn't bothered to bring a coat because I thought Annecy was in Southern France, where it must be warm in the winter. I was wrong. If Budsy were still alive, I'd have brought a coat.

After an agonizing wait alone in the darkness, Gérard opened the door. He was a former monk who'd had some sort of disagreement with his order. Dr. Mérieux hired him as the caretaker.

Gérard was a big man with beefy features, and the porch

light brought out deep wrinkles and creases on his face. He had to bend over to look at me. He used hand signals to wave me back into the wind down the hill into town. I knelt and made begging gestures. Eventually, he relented and guided me in, then pushed me up three flights of stairs and into a chilly garret in the attic. He showed me the bathroom, set out linens and a couple of nice, thick blankets, and went down the stairs. I realized I must have arrived a day early.

Several hours later, I heard a party downstairs, and delicious smells wafted into my room. I lay there, listening to my grumbling stomach, and tried to go to sleep.

The light was too dim to read, so I was staring at the ceiling when Gérard opened the door. He carried a plate heaped with delicious hot food on a tray, a glass, and a bottle of red wine. The following day, I realized I was sticky with sweat and dirt. The shower only had one knob, and the water was freezing. No doubt monks didn't use hot water for their showers. It was more than bracing.

The purpose of our new organization was to help countries build their governments' capacity to fight epidemics. Dr. Mérieux, President of the Mérieux drug company, invited us to use the abbey to get organized.

Charles Mérieux inherited the abbey from his grandfather, Marcel, who assisted Pasteur when he created rabies vaccines. Later, Marcel started his own highly profitable vaccine company. When Charles inherited the family wealth, he created the Fondation Mérieux. He used some of the profits from selling vaccines to his foundation to train people in developing countries' ministries of health.

Manolet and I saw the same need. It seemed odd that the world's malaria experts were all in Europe and the US rather than in countries where scientists dealt with malaria daily. Now that we'd trained hundreds of epidemiologists in developing countries, we wanted to give them a voice.

It turned out that Dr. Mérieux was a good friend of my boss, Steve Thacker. When I told Steve about our idea, he said, "Charles Mérieux will be interested in this." And he was.

The following day, Steve and Barbara Holloway would join me. I was excited to put on my rumpled suit and walk down the stairs to breakfast with the arriving epidemiologists.

Barb was the most humble and effective person I'd ever known. She was a grandmother, though she looked much younger, with long blonde hair and light blue eyes. You can never have too many Barbaras in your life.

We sat at a table in the corner of the dining room. Barbara smiled. "You know, the Europeans and the WHO don't like CDC . . ."

"And Australia," I added.

Steve looked at us with jet-lagged eyes. "Australia, too. So why do you think any of them will work with us?"

I smiled. "Manolet and I are very persuasive."

"I see that."

After breakfast, Gérard and his assistants arranged the furniture in the shape of a big square table so that we were all equal. Manolet, a fine epidemiologist and brilliant manager, led the discussion. He began by projecting an image of an old wooden wagon wheel.

"What holds up the wheel?" he asked reasonably. It was a Zen koan. The answer was the space between the spokes. Nobody had the slightest idea what he was trying to tell us, but the fact that we were equally confused emphasized that we had things in common.

Then a florid, red-haired Irish guy stood up and delivered a flaming denunciation of our proposal, me, CDC, and the US in general. We instantly began calling him the Wild Irish Rose. Guénaël Rodier, the French WHO representative, sat in tight-lipped silence. Australia and Canada asked tense questions dripping with suspicion. I answered my icy audience in what I thought was a reasonable and positive tone. The room exploded when I finally got to the part about how CDC was the first government public health agency to train epidemiologists. I thought I'd get the audience back when I told them CDC would provide start-up funding. Nope. The audience liked this even less. People worried we were trying to take the place of the WHO, and others felt Europe should provide the training, not Americans.

Things went downhill until we finally went to our separate tables in the dining room. Gérard must have sensed things were tense because he introduced us to his liquor before dinner. The taste, somewhere between cough syrup and perfume, was oddly relaxing— but not relaxing enough.

That night, as I stared at the ceiling in my room, I heard a firm knock on my door. It turned out to be Conchy Roces, the Philippine training program director, and an old friend. She was not smiling. "We flew all this way and are spending three days of our lives at this meeting, but if this is just a power play and pissing contest between global players, the directors leave tomorrow." She stood with arms crossed and blazing black eyes.

I didn't need to ask her whether the directors had sent similar envoys to the other major global players. Of course, they had.

The second morning was supposed to be about dividing the tasks, and I was moderating. I had no idea what to say.

I stood before my surly audience and opened my mouth. In a back corner, a craggy man with a pale complexion and wild black hair raised his hand and stood. I'd seen him, but I couldn't remember whether he was David Heymann, a prominent Word Health Organization (WHO) epidemiology expert, or the Ebola expert who tried to get me fired for un-American activities.

He turned out to be David Heymann. He smiled. "Dr. Mérieux asked me to make this announcement. He will provide two million dollars to get you started if you agree to work together and make a global network."

I felt like collapsing with joy. We dedicated the rest of the day to the important business of finding a name. Everybody felt strongly that his idea was the best. Eventually, Mohammed Patel, a Gujarati who had immigrated to Australia, worked his way around the room and collected all the ideas. He then arranged the initials to spell TEPHINET for Training in Public Health Impact and Epidemiology Training Network. Nobody liked it, but we agreed that it was the least undesirable.

The following day, we agreed on a structure. A board of directors chosen by the national programs would administer grants and arrange global meetings. Neither CDC nor WHO was on the board. Then we headed home to present our shiny new global network to our governments. TEPHINET was born. As of 2020, it distributes over $20 million each year to strengthen training programs worldwide.

Guénaël Rodier, director of WHO's Communicable Disease Surveillance and Response Unit, was one of the friendliest and most competent people I met at that meeting. He had brown eyes, short hair, and an unflappable manner. In French-accented English, he told me, "I'm in charge of the International Health Regulations (IHR), and I'm frustrated. We can never make it work because of how it is structured."

I understood. The IHR was a long list of infectious diseases that countries must report yearly to WHO. It was worse than useless because many countries lied to protect their exports. Cholera was a particular problem since many rich countries banned imports of seafood from cholera-endemic countries.

Over sips of Gérard's liquor, Guénaël told me, "I want to improve the health of the people. The way the rules are written, we leave millions of people in developing countries at risk of cholera and take away precious income."

Later, in 2005, Guénaël convinced WHO to get rid of the old system and substitute a requirement for a competent epidemiology unit in each national government. It works much better. I like to think he got part of the idea from his work with FETPs.

Several years later, we met at a WHO meeting in nearby Lyon. The highlight was a dinner during which our Lyonnaise hosts served fantastic food, including slices of pâté de foie gras the size of hamburgers. Nobody could eat this much, and asking for a doggie bag seemed beyond tacky. I rolled half in a napkin and smuggled it out. It made a glorious breakfast spread on fresh baguettes.

TEPHINET still provides millions of dollars a year to FETPs worldwide. When the Spanish FETP hosted a global meeting, I was impressed by their director, Dionisio Herrera, who ran the meeting and raised an extra $50,000 to hold a bang-up conference. He was an attractive guy, a tall, strong man with a fantastic smile. And God, could he dance. I knew several women who lived to dance with him.

Dionisio was from Cuba and once led the Cuban Medical Association. He met Fidel Castro, who sent him on a medical mission to Africa. It says a lot that Dionisio found life in Africa an improvement over that of his native island. He was surprised to learn that life under African dictators was more free and more fun than under Castro. When Dionisio visited Europe, he found that life under capitalist swine in Spain agreed with him. He defected and found a job with the Spanish government, running its epidemiology training program.

Later, Dionisio took over as director of TEPHINET and led

the organization for decades before his tragic death from prostate cancer.

I'll never forget Dionisio's warmth, intellect, and passion.

He was one of the finest people I've ever known. I will always remember his impressive impact on improving people's health worldwide.

CHAPTER 35
SUNSHINE THE CAT

n the year after Budsy died, I looked for her in darkened rooms, in the backyard at night, in dim hallways—everywhere, really. Pictures of her were hanging on half the walls. I'd been married for most of my adult life, and I felt miserable and alone being single.

I flew up to Michigan to consult with my siblings.

My brother Thomas was a practical man. He only drank vodka on the principle that every calorie should carry its weight in bringing pleasure. I admired his self-control. He asked, "Did Budsy ever say she wanted you to stay single?"

"No, she said that she knew I'd remarry."

The corners of his mouth turned up slightly, and his brown eyes looked into mine. "Well? What are you waiting for?"

I couldn't think of what to say.

Thomas ran his fingers through his curly hair. "You ever consider you're torturing yourself because you're afraid to take the plunge again?"

"Yes, Dr. Freud, you may be right."

From his easy chair, he raised his glass in a toast. I clinked my wine glass against it.

Sibyl, his lovely wife, walked in. "Ignore Thomas. You need a woman. The sooner, the better."

She was so right.

My sister, Marty Jo, was even more helpful. She took me on a walk with her yappy little dog, Cinnamon. She'd dyed her hair blonde since she was a teenager, and it would be easier to get the nuclear codes than to find the color underneath.

Marty likes to pretend to be a ditzy blonde. She is neither.

I said, "I've been thinking of what Tom and Sibyl said. God knows I want a relationship. I'm afraid of the months of getting to know a woman. What would it be like to date when you're both middle-aged? The company would be great, but the fights, the anxieties, and the waiting would be tough. It would be terrible if a woman rejected me, but it would be worse if I found I didn't want to marry her after months of courtship. I'd never be able to start over again."

Marty Jo pushed a blonde lock off her forehead. "Isn't there anybody you've known a long time who might be interested in you?"

"I've known a wonderful woman for more than twenty years, but she's sixteen years younger than I am."

Marty grabbed my arm and pulled me closer. "Sixteen years isn't that much for a woman in her forties or fifties. Tell me, please, God, she's single."

"She's single."

"Go call her. Now."

I tracked Shelly Joan Ahmann down and wrote her a letter. She'd lived next door to me in Fort Collins and had held a summer job at the nearby CDC laboratory. I worked there, too, doing bubonic plague research. When Bobbie, my first wife, left me, I was distraught and terribly lonely. Shelly's saintly mother took me in. She and Shelly babysat, and June tried to convert me to Catholicism. After work each day, I found myself walking next door to sit on the sliding couch on her back porch.

We drank water or iced tea and admired June's carefully tended flowers. Sometimes Shelly joined us.

June had an old, decaying horse-drawn carriage covered in morning-glory vines in her back garden, a wonderful touch. Statues of Mary and Jesus watched over the flowers. June was a Catholic in the truest and best sense of the word. She lived frugally and volunteered to help the poor or patients in nursing homes. She befriended the poor—a Good Samaritan.

Shelly followed her mother's example. One of the nicest things June did for Shelly was to raise money to send her to Latin America each summer with an organization called *Amigos de las Americas*. In the summers, Shelly helped health workers in Central America by giving oral polio immunizations to kids. I was amazed to learn she had spent summers in remote villages in Venezuela and Honduras. One summer, she worked with the Sandinistas in Nicaragua, teaching peasant families to read and write. The Ahmanns were an impressive family.

After I moved east to be near Bobbie and the boys, June and Shelly sent me Christmas cards each year. When Shelly went to college, she began sending me her own cards. One year, she wrote, "I want to be a tropical medicine doctor like you." That felt good.

She studied biology and took premed classes. One summer, she wrote to me, asking whether I knew of a summer job. By then, I lived in New York City. AIDS had just emerged, and I was beginning a study comparing the white blood cells of hemodialysis patients with those of early AIDS patients, and I needed a helper. Shelly took the job.

Two years later, she went to the University of Colorado School of Medicine. In her Christmas card, she asked me for advice.

I wrote her, "When you get to the clinical years, take surgery first. It's a nightmare, and you'll want to get it out of the way before you take the courses that will prepare you for tropical medicine."

The following year, she wrote, "Thanks for the advice on surgery. It's so great to reach in and take away somebody's pain and maybe save their life. You have to be smart and skilled. I'm working hard and hope to get a surgical residency."

The following year, I wrote a short card. "Merry Christmas. I thought you wanted to save the world. It looks like you settled for taking out a few of its parts."

I didn't reply to her Christmas letters after that.

Eighteen years later, I took my sister and brother's advice and tracked her down. She was Chief of Surgery at the Northern Navajo Medical Center on a reservation in New Mexico. I sent her an email, she wrote back, and we began exchanging messages.

Finally, I found some courage and invited her to visit me, and she agreed. I called her to make plans. "I'll wait for you at the gate. I'll have a book. I look older now, with less hair and a graying beard. I hope you're still coming."

"I'm coming," she said. "I look the same." And she did.

In those days, you could wait at the arrival gates. I tried to keep my eyes from showing the need and anxiety roiling inside. I missed Budsy, and I couldn't help but look at the passing crowd in case she might be there.

Then Shelly walked off the plane, tall and blonde in jeans and a T-shirt. She wore a well-used backpack. I was far too nervous to attempt to kiss her hello, which was just as well because I could feel sweat building up on my upper lip.

So much had happened since we last met that we chatted up a storm all the way home. I almost forgot my aching need to be with her until we pulled up in the driveway. "Let me show you the house. Let's start with your room." I led her to the spare bedroom. I felt a sharp tug as I realized Budsy had put a portrait of herself on the wall. She had put up pictures of herself on every wall. I'd been living with her ghost in this museum for so long that I'd ceased to notice.

Shelly slid her backpack off and dropped it on the bed. "Let's see the rest of the house," she said, and smiled sweetly.

We found that Sunshine, Budsy's scruffy yellow tomcat, had left a gnawed dead bird on the couch in the basement.

Shelly and I headed upstairs to the more civilized living room.

CHAPTER 36
THE HOLY CHILIS

T hat evening, we retired to the living room and drank red wine with our feet on the glass coffee table. We looked out into the night at the steep, weedy backyard, faintly lit by the moon and my neighbor's security lights. Later, she looked down at the coffee table's glass top, then bent down to examine it closely. She pointed to a red stain. "Looks like somebody's lipstick."

"It's a wine stain." I pointed to my glass.

She scraped the stain with her fingernail and tasted it. "Probably right." She straightened to look at me across the table. Her whole face smiled.

In the morning, I got up, went to the bathroom, and saw in the mirror that I had a big, happy, goofy smile. I made a pot of coffee and waited for Shelly to awaken.

For most of the following year, we both wore smiles. It was impossible not to.

I obsessed over the color of her eyes. CDC published a weekly newsletter, the *Morbidity and Mortality Weekly Report*. I went to the office and sat down with an artist who helped me match my memory of Shelly's eyes on the color charts. They are somewhere between cerulean and azure blue.

When she flew back to New Mexico, I emailed her a haiku every morning we were apart. Sonnets eluded me. I'm a seventeen-syllable kind of guy. She wrote back with poems, including a few sonnets. We talked each night and alternated weekly visits.

I'd fly into Albuquerque, the nearest big airport, then drive north through the desert for several hours. This world was brown in various shades. The only green was little strips of cottonwoods around the narrow rivers.

I'd driven through bleak Western deserts to investigate people with bubonic plague. From the airport, I took the arrow-straight road from Albuquerque past huge mesas looming over the desert. To the north, the landscape was immense, empty, and oppressive. There were always rocks piled around the base of each mesa. Later, I learned that the ancient rock formations were melting away, eroding over life-times and centuries. For the first time, I understood that we exist in the vastness of geological time.

Towns were many miles apart, and most were named for their most salient features: Red Rock, Black Rock, etc.

Shelly lived in Shiprock, a sleepy town in the shadow of the great rock. The Spanish thought it looked like a sailing ship. Since ancient times, the Navajos have called it *Tsé Bit'a'í*, which means "the winged rock." Don't ask how it is pronounced. Navajo is such a difficult tonal language that in World War II, the army used Navajo soldiers for battlefield radio communications in Asia. They were called the code talkers, and the Japanese never figured out their language.

The first night I visited Shelly, I found she lived in a little row of connected houses. It was like married student housing in college, with a kitchen, bathroom, two bedrooms, and a common area with a dining table and a big picture window. She had a big golden retriever named Litso, Navajo for "yellow."

Her picture window faced the Shiprock. It's about twice as

tall as the Empire State Building and looks like a dinosaur with immense wings. It was amazing watching the morning light reveal its contours.

Often she drove us out into the desert. We gained altitude quickly. After a few miles, the ditch by the road was heaped with snow. Shelly hit the brakes. "Litso loves snow." She opened the door, and he galumphed out and jumped into the snow up to his belly, then threw snow up with his paws and disappeared as he rolled under the surface, only to pop his head up and plow ahead. It felt great watching him—a contact high.

Eventually, we drove back down into the desert, and the three of us started walking across the sandy rock. Shelly suddenly stopped and led us out to the entrance of a canyon. It was too steep for Litso, and he perched nervously, looking into the shadow of the steep path.

Shelly said, "If he comes down, we'll have to carry him out." She tied his leash to a rock, and we headed down into what looked like a big cave and walked for a while. Suddenly we emerged into sunlight. Tufts of grass and scattered stones covered the canyon floor. High up a far wall, she pointed out a line of cliff dwellings clinging near the top. I could imagine the ancient Indians looking down on us. Nobody knows what they called themselves, so people use the Navajo word *Anasazi*, which means "the Old Ones." Somebody had placed a wooden ladder up to the buildings. I assumed it was modern, a replacement for the wooden ones the Anasazis must have made. If enemies appeared, they'd pull the ladders up. The buildings were made of rectangular, light-brown bricks and stood along the broad ledge.

She said, "The Indians raised corn and other vegetables on fertile soil on top of nearby mesas. I love that they were peaceful farmers," she said.

We climbed off the ladder and stood in silence among little adobe buildings. It felt like a holy place. Desiccated little corn cobs lay around. They made us feel the Anasazi were nearby. It amazed me that visitors left the empty buildings and the corncobs alone over the centuries. They must have felt it was sacred, too.

Later, *National Geographic* magazine had an article about archeologists who studied bones left scattered among the ruins. The bones showed signs they had been boiled in a pot.

Another weekend, she drove me out into the desert to the Church of the Holy Dirt in Chimayo. Like everything else in New Mexico, it was hours across the scrubby desert. As the miles and hours ticked by, I remembered stories about psychos who take people to the remote desert and kill them. After an hour, I said, "Stop, please. I have to pee."

"There are no trees or bushes," Shelly said through pursed lips.

Suddenly, I felt like somebody was squeezing my bladder. "There are also no people. We haven't seen anybody for at least an hour."

"Just hold it. On a busy surgery day, I might not pee between breakfast and coming home from work. Don't be a baby."

"I'll try." A biting edge of anger snaked its way up from my belly and into my chest. I wondered if I'd survive jumping out of the car and rolling. However, this wouldn't do if I wanted to marry her, so I crossed my legs.

We finally arrived at a little compound of adobe buildings. The biggest was the church. Signs said the spring dried up hundreds of years ago, and no holy water remained for communions. A missionary priest found a crucifix sticking out of the sand where the spring had been. He rescued it and placed it in a position of honor on the altar. The next day, the cross was back in the sandpit. The priest realized something was special about the sand and poured a handful on a sick parishioner, who was instantly cured.

Seeing a bathroom by the church door, I was cured, too.

As I stepped out, Shelly picked up the story. "Eventually, so many people made the pilgrimage that the parishioners tore the church down and rebuilt a larger version right over what they now called 'the Holy Sandpit.'"

"You've got to see this," she said and steered me into a large, dim room filled with canes, crutches, old medicine bottles, and glasses. Her delighted smile lit up the room. "These guys are going to put doctors out of business.

I said, "Shells, do you know what Émile Zola said about people getting healed at Lourdes?"

She put a hand on her hip. "Enlighten me."

"He said, 'The road to Lourdes is littered with crutches but no wooden legs.'"

She looked at me with tolerant irritation. "Here's a plastic bag." She led me around behind the altar and past a sign that said, Holy Sand. No Playing. We each filled a quart bag.

She dropped twenty bucks into an offering box and said, "Let's check out the Holy Chili stand."

The stand stood next to the church, curtained by white sheets spray-painted with Day-Glo pictures of Jesus with the Sacred Heart. Vastly amused, I asked the tall Hispanic guy inside to come out and snap a photo of Shelly and me with the sign. I thought it was a joke. It wasn't. Turning the other cheek, the guy walked out and snapped the picture. "Do you want any chilies, or was that it?" he asked crabbily.

We bought a couple of strings of dried chilies and headed home. They turned out to be flavorful and spicy. If we ever go back, I'll buy some more.

I put my bag of Holy Dirt in the drawer of my bedside table. Over the decades, it's leaked out and distributed itself throughout the house.

Perhaps it's a coincidence, but I've had a lot of good luck since.

CHAPTER 37
THE NOTHING FESTIVAL

My next visit to Shelly after the Holy Chili adventure Shelly was full of surprises. She showed me a cupboard that contained a dozen plastic martini glasses. "I got them for Jack and his fellows."

"Should I be jealous of Jack and his jolly good fellows?"

Wry face and frown. "No, you bonehead. Jack is a plastic surgery professor at Emory School of Medicine. Twice a year, he flies a few of his fellows and residents out, and they do plastic surgery on kids with harelips and whatnot. I make a big dinner for them." She eyed me thoughtfully.

"He pays the fares for all of them?"

"No, he flies them out in his private plane. It's a big one-prop job. He's won some races with it."

"Well, now I know what kind of doctor I should've been."

She ignored me.

"After they fix the kids, he flies the fellows up to Telluride, where he has a big lodge, and they ski."

"He ever fly you up?"

"Nope, but he lets me stay there sometimes. He's agreed to let the two of us use it next weekend. It's just over the Colorado border from New Mexico. We're going to the Nothing Festival."

It turned out that the town set a festival nearly every weekend to draw visitors. They didn't celebrate this one weekend so that the locals could enjoy it without crowds. We would join the locals and take some quiet hikes.

Shelly kissed my cheek. "I want to show you some of the most beautiful things in the world. They're little flowers that grow above the tree line. We have to go early in the morning." Later, I would regret not asking why.

We drove north to Jack's cabin, went out for a great dinner, and slept in. So much for an early start. As we walked into a restaurant for breakfast, I picked up a copy of the morning's *Telluride Daily Planet* from an empty table. A full page was dedicated to horoscopes. A big headline said, "No More Crème Brûlée, Pisces." Even though I'm a Sagittarius, it seemed like good advice.

Shelly looked over her scrambled eggs. "Hey, we've got to get going. It rains up there nearly every afternoon."

"I hope there's no lightning."

"Not a problem. I brought slickers for both of us.

"I'm worried about lightning. Remember, I was electro-cuted and almost had to have my arm amputated."

She lay cash on the table to pay for breakfast. "Better head up right away, then. Lightning doesn't strike twice in the same place, right?"

"It was a short circuit in Africa," I grumped.

She took my hand and led me out into the sunshine past the line of people waiting for tables.

It was a short drive to the trailhead, which began beside a historic power station that powered a nearby gold mine. Electricity is my bane and passion—I love computers and making robots with my kids.

Shelly led me up the trail, which became cooler and sunnier as the trees and bushes disappeared. We began to see little blue-gray pasqueflower clumps along the path. Some petals caught the exact shade of Shelly's eyes in the sunlight.

We passed the tree line, and the landscape turned rocky and bare. Little rodents began popping out of cracks among the rocks, whistling sharply, giving us nasty looks, then ducking down.

Shelly said, "Those are pikas, little mouselike guys. They only live above the tree line."

"Huh," I said. The thin air was getting to me.

She walked me across a rocky moonscape to a small valley with scattered patches of scrubby alpine tundra, short, brown, dark-green grass, and little flat bushes, maybe six inches high. Some had cushions of tiny, light-blue forget-me-nots. I was tempted to pick some, but Shelly reached out and pulled my hand away.

"This is a delicate ecosystem. It's against the law to walk on it."

"Right," I said, "Sorry." A cold wind picked up and sucked the warmth away. Just like that, the sky clouded over.

She grabbed my hand. "Storm's coming! We've got to get down. We can put on the raincoats later."

We ran, holding hands like Hansel and Gretel. I tripped a couple of times but stayed on my feet. A massive bolt of green lightning struck about twenty yards away. The air vibrated with a loud crack.

"Shelly, lightning strikes the tallest thing around, and that's us."

"I know, you wimp. Let's duck under this tall rock."

There wasn't enough space under the rock, so we huddled beside it and tried to avoid the stinging rain. The rock was about ten feet taller than we were, which was good. On the other hand, it drew lightning. We couldn't talk because the rain and thunder drowned us out. Shelly scanned the mountaintop looking for another rock. We were both cold and shivering, but Shelly was focused. I was glad she was an experienced mountain climber.

I can't say how long we crouched there. It seemed like

eons. Even after the rain quieted, we sat silently, staring into the gloomy haze. Shelly had an arm around me and gave me a little shake. I stood up and realized my bottom was soaking and freezing from sitting in an icy puddle. We held hands down the long, dank, slippery trail to the car. I never looked more forward to a hot bath and a nap. I had something important to say.

The next day, Shelly took me to a little monument near another old generator. It proudly documented that Telluride was the first city west of the Continental Divide to have alternating electric current. Quite an achievement.

It probably had a lot to do with Nicola Tesla's setting up his laboratory in nearby Colorado Springs. The city power company agreed to provide him with space and unlimited electricity to research transmitting current through the atmosphere or soil without wires. He built a 142-foot-high Tesla coil and began making giant bolts of what he called "artificial lightning." Tesla's theories about conducting electricity through atmospheric and geological layers proved correct.

For someone who's been severely shocked, vacationing in a place with lightning in the history and air was not my first choice, but it appealed to Shelly, so it appealed to me.

That night, we went to an expensive restaurant and sat on the balcony. It had to be perfect because I had an important question to ask.

We started with vodka martinis in honor of Jack and his gaggle of plastic surgeons.

In the darkness, Shelly's eyes shone across the table. "Do you think we should have anything else to drink? I'm feeling it already."

"As your internist, I'd advise beer or wine, depending on our entrees."

We both ordered fish, so we got a bottle of Pinot Grigio.

Afterward, she had decaf with her dessert, and so did I—and a glass of VSOP cognac. It was excellent.

At last, I could bring myself to ask my question. "Shelly, will you marry me?"

She looked blankly across the table and said nothing. The starry glint in her eyes had disappeared halfway through the wine. Now they showed nothing.

Seconds ticked by. She was silent. She seemed to be falling asleep. I got up, walked around the table, and knelt on both knees. People were looking, which would make it more embarrassing if she refused.

"Shelly Joan Ahmann, will you please marry me?" I tried not to look like I was begging, which I was.

Her face looked down on me like a full moon seen through fog. She asked, "Does this mean we're engaged?"

"Only if you say yes."

"Yes, yes, of course, yes. Now let's go home and get to bed."

I can't remember if the other diners applauded. Whether they did or not, they should have.

CHAPTER 38
THE WEDDING VASE

N ow that we were engaged, it was time to plan the wedding. I became alarmed when Shelly said, "I've found the perfect place for our wedding. It's an event barn just over the Colorado border."

"You want to get married in a barn? I've been married in a church and a hospital, but a barn seems extreme."

"Don't worry. It's just outside Durango."

"Where they used to have gunfights?"

She smiled. "There's a joke. 'How do you become a millionaire in Durango?'"

"Rob the stagecoach?"

"Bring two million."

"Fine. Getting married in a barn sounds like a great idea."

"I thought you'd say that," she agreed.

The red barn turned out to be a beautiful venue.

T he ceremony would be held outside against the backdrop of the La Plata Mountains. Blessedly, I had nothing to do with the arrangements except finding a minister to wed us. Colorado is exceptionally reasonable about who performs marriages. Couples can have a licensed minister or marry themselves by filling out a registration form. In one case, a humorous couple was married by their dog. I was much more conservative and chose a new-age priestess named Crystal, who had a certificate from an Internet church.

I agreed with Shelly that we should include elements from the charming Navajo wedding tradition. This was not, of course, a Navajo wedding.

I hadn't expected so many people, but Shelly was much beloved in the medical community. All her relatives were there as well. My family was there in force, too. My father has terrible air sickness, so flying to Colorado was out of the question. However, my saintly sister came to the rescue and loaded mom and dad on a train for the long trip.

By this time, dad, who had once been a benign patriarch, had morphed into a full-blown curmudgeon. They arrived on time, my sister and mother looking the worse for wear, but game. Dad told stories about how he taught disrespectful whippersnappers lessons on the train, waving his cane like a rapier.

My sons, Alex and Daniel, were there, too. Alex wore a tasteful suit, and Daniel sported a red jacket embroidered with Chinese dragons. Tom Keever, my best friend and former Shakespearean actor, also was there. After decades of starving on actors' wages, he tried technical directing (TD) and found that he liked it. Being a TD paid better, too. He opened a checking account and joined the mainstream economy. Tom always carried a clipboard, pencil, and a thick sheaf of paper, even after he earned a master's degree in theater history at Columbia and began teaching. It's surprising how often the clipboard turned out to be helpful.

The night before the ceremony, the Internet priestess didn't show up for the rehearsal.

Keever rose to the occasion. "My family wanted me to be a minister. They'll be happy to hear I married at least one couple."

Shelly gave him a copy of the service. He snapped it firmly onto his clipboard.

Tom's years of acting showed through. He was incredible. His melodious voice projected out over the prairie in a warm, ceremonious, perfect pitch. Thank God Crystal didn't answer her phone.

The following day, the sky was bright and so clear you could make out details of the mountains in the background. All went well as I marched down the aisle and stood proudly with my brother Thomas before the congregation. Shelly missed her cue. A minute crept by, then another. I heard a hiss, and Thomas turned back and disappeared into the barn. I stood alone, facing Keever and the mountains. Keever raised his eyebrows, and I made a face. Birds traced figures above us. Bees visited the bridal flowers. Tom's eyes told me nothing of what was going on behind me. I contemplated a future even more alone than before.

Finally, Shelly's mother and Thomas led Shelly forward.

Keever switched seamlessly into the service. Shelly's mom brought us a big, flat, round Navajo wedding basket, traditionally inhabited by good spirits. The concentric design always includes a little straight path where the spirits can come out if they want to visit their friends.

Two little piles of blue corn pollen sat on the basket. I reached in first, took a little pollen ball, and pushed it into her mouth. It was surprising how hard it was to get the sticky corn pollen into her mouth without making a mess. She winced, smiled, then fed me some.

Navajos make unique wedding vases with two necks, one for the bride and one for the groom. Before the ceremony, you fill it with water to wash the pollen from your hands. We practiced this the night before.

When it came time to wash off the corn pollen, Thomas held up a plain white pitcher. As Shelly poured the cold water onto my fingers, I barely noticed that it had only one neck. Keever pronounced us man and wife, and the audience surrounded us with kisses, hugs, and good wishes.

After the ceremony, my mother told us how beautiful Shelly looked. "Shelly, when you were late, in my mind's eye, I could see you running away across the plains into the mountains."

"No, Betty, not a chance," Shelly said graciously.

"That's good because we've taken him back after two wives, and we're not taking him back again. He's yours now."

Shelly smiled beautifully. Since then, we've been married for more than 23 of the happiest years of my life.

t turned out that the wedding vase had melted. It had worked fine the night before, but the water had softened it, and the bottom turned to mud by morning. We bought it at a trading post, which neglected to tell us that the pot hadn't been fired. It was just dried mud.

While I stood alone before the crowd, Shelly called Thomas into the barn. She looked fiercely at him and said, "Get another pitcher now." Fortunately, the barn had a full kitchen, and he quickly found one.

A few days later, we visited the trading post where Shelly bought the pot. The grizzled Anglo manager said, "Tourists know they shouldn't put water in them. Nobody's ever returned one."

Shelly glared. "I live here, and I doubt people who live far away feel like calling you when their pots melt."

He gave us a replacement but refused to provide us with one that had been fired.

· · ·

We honeymooned in the Monteverde Cloud Forest of Costa Rica, home of the gorgeously resplendent and large quetzal birds, measuring about a foot and a half long, with impressive two-foot-long bluish-green tails.

During mating season, males' tails grow to four feet long. The ancient Aztecs and Mayans viewed the bird as sacred to Quetzalcoatl, the Feathered Serpent god.

Shelly, a passionate birdwatcher, chose the place. I booked us into the honeymoon suite of a little hotel near the rain-forest entrance. A large jacuzzi filled the room. Explicit statues stood at each corner, but the pièce de résistance was the giant mural of jaguars courting and mating on all four walls. There was no danger that a guest wouldn't understand the mechanics of the physical side of marriage.

Each day, we hiked deeper into the darkness of the forest paths seeking quetzals. It was dim beneath the canopy, with cold water dripping down into the chilly dankness. We could occasionally see little brown birds darting about. We assumed that if we got away from the crowds of other tourists and penetrated miles into the forest, it would reveal its secrets. Not so.

On our final morning there, we pulled into the parking lot, and a guy walked up to us and offered to guide us for half a day for $15. He was well-dressed and intelligent-looking, so we agreed.

"If you want to see quetzals," he began in the voice of a genial professor, "you need to know what they like to eat in each season."

Annoyed, I said, "So, what do they eat this season?"

"Wild avocados."

"How far do we have to go to find them?" Shelly asked politely.

"About 20 feet," he said, pointing to a little tree in the lot. "The fruit is the big, avocado-shaped berries."

"How long do we have to wait here before we might see one?"

"Look over there. I see another across the lot. The park planted the trees here to attract the birds."

Humbled and respectful, I began snapping pictures.

"Are there other interesting animals in the forest? Can you show them to us?"

"There are animals in the forest, but you can't see them. If you'd taken the forest path, you'd have known that instantly."

"Yeah," I said, "I know what you mean."

"If you'll give me a ride home, I'll show you some more."

We hopped in our rental car and rolled down the windows, then soon afterward heard a piercing, loud grating sound, like a giant rusty door opening.

"Stop here," he said. "It's a three-wattled bellbird. If we sit still, we can probably see one."

"You're pulling our leg, right?" I asked.

He and Shelly pointed to a big red and white bird about 20 feet away. It had two long black wattles on one side and only one on the other. Why such a ridiculous-looking bird evolved with these unbalanced wattles, I don't know. Neither did our professor, an unusual event. He seemed to know everything else about the animals and plants.

Ten minutes later, he motioned for me to stop and back up. He pointed to a tree. "See that three-toed sloth?" It took a minute, but as my eyes adjusted, I could see it.

"I didn't know there were green ones," I said. "No wonder they're so hard to find."

It's humid up there, and the sloths rarely move, so algae grow on them. Symbiosis."

"Shelly shouted, "Look, it's got a baby on its back!"

Terrified it would disappear, I fumbled for the camera,

and the lens cap fell with a noise that sounded like a bomb going off. However, the animal didn't move. What else would you expect from a sloth?

The naturalist invited us into his cottage. It was filled with books and his hand-drawn sketches. He had a bachelor's degree in biology and was trying to raise money to get a master's. I felt a pinch in my heart at the unfairness. If this guy were from the US, he'd be teaching in a famous university, not living on $15 a day, including saving to pay for classes.

I gave him $30.

Now I wish I'd given him a thousand.

THE END

EPILOGUE

S teve Thacker, who appointed me Director of the Division of International Health in CDC's Epidemiology Program Office, was an outstanding man, intelligent, thoughtful, and passionate. He was the conscience of CDC, and everyone from the CDC director down asked for his advice on ethics. Steve kept the agency from deviating from its public health mission or being politicized. His early death was a tragedy for all of us and people all over the world.

Steve didn't have much money for FETPs, so I raised five to ten million dollars a year from donors, primarily USAID. I led teams that started new national and regional programs that serve more than half the world's population, including China, India, Japan, Central Asia, Kenya, and Central America.

I made many friends at CDC. Ed Maes was a great Associate Director for Science. For some reason, women seemed attracted to him. I remember one night we went to the Bolshoi Ballet in Moscow. Notably, they serve vodka in graduate cylinders, like in chemistry labs. After the show ended, we joined the crowd pouring out into the dark streets. Two gorgeous women on horses swept up to us, and one gestured she'd like Ed to climb up on her with her. Oddly, the other didn't ask me to climb up. Ed, a gentle and genuinely good man, stuck with me.

Terry Chorba ran our office in Central Asia when the Soviet Union fell apart. When they say "central heating" there, they mean one furnace for the whole town. Terry used to email us pictures of him typing on his computer with gloves on.

Terry introduced me to Michal Favorov, who had been in charge of the medical clinics at the Moscow Olympics. He got kicked out of Russia for consorting with foreigners. Michael built up the programs in the former Soviet Republics in Central Asia, and we had many adventures together.

Peter Nsubuga, my Ugandan branch chief, had a great sense of humor and built our African programs to cover nearly the entire continent.

Henry Walke, another branch chief, supervised the Brazilian program and married a beautiful graduate. He spoke with a soft southern accent, and was embarrassed when I read Shelby Foote's history of the civil war and learned that his forebear, also named Henry Walke, was a captain in the Union army who sailed past the embattled southern fortress at Vicksburg and fired artillery into the fort allowing Grant to capture it. As a northerner, I am grateful to both Walkes.

When we started the Chinese FETP, the Minister of Health invited me to a celebratory banquet. She sat me next to her, and we chatted as people passed dozens of delicacies on a big lazy Susan in the center of the table. She delicately took a cherry tomato with her chopsticks and popped it into her mouth. I was delighted at the chance to show off my skills. Unfortunately, my tomato slipped off my sticks and rolled over the tablecloth to the floor. Quickly, I reached for my chopsticks to pick up another. As I brought it to my lips, it fell, too. I watched it bounce and roll across the tablecloth and into the minister's lap. She reached into the bowl, picked up a tomato, and popped it into her mouth. Then she reached into the bowl, took out a cherry tomato, and held it to my lips.

She was an extraordinarily gracious host.

Branch Chief Sharon McDonnell was incredibly productive. When she was in charge of diseases caused by iron imbalances, Time magazine called her "The Iron Maiden." Another Branch Chief, Rubina Imtiaz, negotiated several new programs, including India. For 20 years, CDC tried and failed to help the Indians set up a Field Epidemiology Training Program. Rubina succeeded. Her husband, Jim Andersen, became the first director of TEPHINET.

After 9/11, CDC was reorganized, and my division was moved from under Steve Thacker to the Center for Global Health, where my new bosses promptly replaced me with one of their friends and made me a science officer. I enjoyed it, but still, I missed working in the field and fell into an awful depression. I got it under control with lots of help from Shelly and my therapists.

I couldn't wait to retire, left on my 65th birthday, and went to work on this memoir and RightSize, a statistical computer program to calculate survey sample sizes.

Shelly and I adopted two wonderful sisters from Ethiopia. They are both strikingly beautiful. There is a reason people call Ethiopians "the beautiful people."

As with my two boys from my marriage to Bobbie, they are sources of joy, frustration, and worry. When we met, Leila, whose name means "Night Beauty," was five. She's completed two years in fashion design at the oddly-named SCAD. It stands for Savannah College of Arts and Design.

ZuZu, whose Ethiopian name means "Little Butter," is in her third year studying integrated design, whatever that is, at Parsons College of Design in Manhattan. My older son Alex is writing TV scripts and caring for our grandchildren, Ry and

Casey, in Los Angeles. His brother, Daniel, lives with his lovely Japanese wife, Kumi, in Boston.

Most of my friends from the Philippines are in the text, but one, the vivacious Vikki Delosreyes, became Training Officer years after I left. We became friends on my visits. I love to watch her give speeches and lectures. She literally jumps with joy. Often. I hope many graduates follow in her footsteps.

There are so many more friends and stories I couldn't fit in or can't remember. They enriched my life immeasurably. And I am immeasurably grateful for all the opportunities and adventures life has given all of us.

ACKNOWLEDGMENTS

Professor Carol Lee Lorenzo, my fiery muse and mentor, stood by me for the 12 years it took to write this volume. She forced me to keep writing until each chapter was up to snuff. I also thank my many fellow students who provided inspiration and excellent advice.

Over the years, I worked for the US Centers for Disease Control and Prevention (CDC), the Rockefeller Foundation, the US Agency for International Development, and the World Health Organization. Tom Monath, Steve Thacker, and Manolet Dayrit were wonderful mentors and models. I thank them for making my work possible. Murray Trostle of USAID was a great partner. In addition to the funding, I learned much from him.

I am especially grateful to Guénaël Rodier of the World Health Organization. He helped organize TEPHINET and revised the International Health Regulations to require that countries have field epidemiology competencies.

Shelly Joan Ahmann, my saintly wife, supported me in every way through this long and challenging process. My years with her have been among the happiest of my life. And she has the most beautiful smile.

Bobbie White, my first wife, corrected and proofread many chapters and produced a timeline to help keep things in order.

My niece and right-wing firebrand, Carrie Severino, read most of the book to her children and sent helpful comments. Steve Reccia, sculptor and intellectual, reviewed the manuscript also. Rod Ellis, who maintains the OHS graduate website helped let grads know about the book. Sheri Carmon proofread the paperback and helped me fix a bunch of problems.

Ms. Boznango, my high school English and writing teacher, believed in me. She made all the difference.

BIBLIOGRAPHY

Learn more about Mark White's Investigations.

Nsubuga P, White M, Fontaine R, Simone P. Training programmes for field
 epidemiology
Lancet 2008;371:630-631.

Barrett D, White M. Ethical pandemic planning (letter). *Hastings Center
 Report.* 2008;38:4.

Traicoff DA, Walke HT, Jones, DS, Gogstad EK, Imtiaz R, White, ME. Repli-
 cating success: developing a standard FETP curriculum. *Public Health
 Reports* 2008 supp;123:28-34.

White ME, Guibert-Herrera JD, Lim-Quizon MC. Joined up public health
 initiatives. *Lancet* 2006;367:1301-1302.

Nsubuga P, White ME, Thacker S, et al. Public health surveillance: a tool for
 targeting and monitoring interventions. In Jamison DT, Breman JG,
 Measham, et al. (eds.) *Disease control priorities in developing countries, second
 edition.* New York: Oxford University Press, 2006. p 997-1015.

McDonnell SM, Bolton P, Sunderland N, Bellows B, White M, Noji E. The role
 of epidemiologists in armed conflict. *Emerging Themes in Epidemiology* 2004,
 1:4 (7 October 2004)

Sandhu HS, Thomas C, Nsubuga P, White ME. A global network for early
 warning and response to infectious diseases and bioterrorism: *American
 Journal of Public Health* 2003; 93:1640-42.

White ME, McDonnell SM, Werker DH, Cardenas VM, Thacker, ST. Partner-
 ships in international applied epidemiology training and service, 1975-
 2001. *American Journal of Epidemiology.* 2001; 154:993-999.

White ME, McDonnell S. Public health surveillance in low and middle-income
 countries. In: Teutsch SM, Churchill RE, eds. *Principles and practice of public
 health surveillance.* 2nd ed. New York, NY; Oxford University Press, 2000.

Spence RJS, Antionios Pomonas, Baxter PJ, Coburn AW, White ME, Dayrit
 MM, FETP Team. In Newhall CG and Puongbayan RS (eds.) *Fire and mud:*

eruptions and lahars of Mount Pinatubo, Philippines. Seattle: University of Washington Press, 1996. P 1055-1062.

Surmieda MR, Lopez JM, Abad-Viola G, et al. Surveillance in evacuation camps after the eruption of Mt. Pinatubo, Philippines. *MMWR CDC Surveill Summ* 1992;41(SS-4):9–12.

Lim-Quizon MC, Benabaye RM, White FM, Dayrit MM, White ME. Cholera in metropolitan Manila: foodborne transmission via street vendors. *Bull WHO* 1994;72:745-749.

Roces MC, White ME, Dayrit MM, Durkin ME. Risk factors for injuries due to the 1990 earthquake in Luzon, Philippines. *Bull WHO* 1992;70:509-14.

Miranda MEG, White ME, Dayrit MM, Hayes CG, Ksiazek TG, Burans JP. Seroepidemiological study of filovirus related to Ebola in the Philippines. (Letter) *Lancet* 1991;337:425-426.

Rayray RU, Salva EP, Pastor NI, White ME, Dayrit MM. Outbreak of febrile gastroenteritis in a Five Star Hotel in Metro Manila. *JPMA* 1991;66:180-185.

Magboo, FP, Abellanosa I, Tayag E, Pascual ML, Magpantay R, Abad G, Surmeida MR, White ME, Dayrit, MM. Fireworks injuries in Metro Manila during the 1991 New Year's Celebration. *JPMA* 1991;67:68-71.

Sadang RA, Zacarias NS, Pastor NI, Catan R, White ME, Dayrit MM. Injuries after new years celebration seen at the National Orthopedic Hospital. *JPMA* 1991;66:164-169.

Lopez JM, Sadang RA, Brizuela MB, Bautista NB, White ME, Dayrit MM. Malaria in Quarry Mining Companies, San Ildelfonso, Bulacan. *Phil J Micro Infect Dis* 1991;20:6-12.

Gopez I, Manoff S, White ME, Dayrit MM. Meningococcal disease outbreak in San Jose Ildefonso, Bulacan. *Phil J Infect Dis* 1991; 20:6-12.

Gavino RR, Salva EP, Gregorio SP, White ME, Dayrit MM. A report of ether vapor poisoning in an underground water storage tank in Makati, Metro Manila. *JPMA* 1990;65:343-344.

Pastor NI, White ME, Dayrit MM. Formalin in fish: investigation of the fish preservative panic of 1987. *JPMA* 1990;65:330-333.

Salva EP, Conanan EC, Quizon MCL, Trocio CT, White ME, et al. Meningococcal disease in Southeastern Mindanao. *JPMA* 1990;65: 336-342.

Guerrero ET, Dayrit MM, White ME. Epidemiological investigation of alcohol-related encephalopathy in Metro Manila. *JPMA* 1989;65: 199-203.

Gregorio SP, Lofranco VS, Auza C, White F, Merin J, Dayrit MM, White ME. Dengue fever outbreak in Cebu. *Phil J Micro Infect Dis* 1989;18:16-20.

Pastor NI, Gopez I, Quizon CL, Bautista N, White ME, Dayrit MM. Epidemic of paralytic shellfish poisoning in the Philippines, 1988-1989. In: Hallegraeff GM, Maclean JL, eds.*Biology, epidemiology, and management of Pyrodinium red tides*. Philippines: International Center for Aquatic Resources Management, 1989:279- 286.

Conanan EC, Dayrit MM, Flores BB, White ME. Typhoid fever pseudoepidemic in Oroquieta City: lessons in the inappropriate use of the Widal test. *JPMA* 1989;65:205-209.

White ME. Footsteps of cholera in Manila. *Phil J Micro Infect Dis* 1989;18:10-11.

Benabaye RS, Guerrero ET, White ME. Measles outbreak in Tawangan Benguet. *JPMA* 1988;64:7-10.

Lofranco VS, Gregorio SP, White ME. A waterborne outbreak of typhoid fever in Baliwag Bulacan. *Phil J Micro Infect Dis* 1988; 17:9-12.

White ME, Butler T, Poland JD. Plague and tularemia pneumonia. pp. 93-109. In: Weinstein L, Fields BN, eds. *Seminars in infectious disease*. New York: Thieme-Stratton, 1983:93-109.

White ME, Russo B. An outbreak of methicillin-resistant <u>Staphylococcus</u> <u>aureus</u>. *J Hosp Infect* 1984;2:Suppl 135-143.

White ME, Rosenbaum RJ, Canfield TM, Poland JD. Plague in a neonate and a discussion of plague in the pediatric age group. Am J Dis Child 1981; 135:418-419.

White ME, Plague. In: Conn HC, ed. Conn's current therapy Philadelphia: Saunders, 1980:52-53.

White ME, Gordon DM, Poland JD, Barnes AM. Recommendations for the control of Yersinia pestis infections. Infect Control 1980;1:324-329.

Morens DM, Woodall JP, Lopez-Correa R, Sather GE, White ME, Chester TJ, Moore CG, Kappus KD. Dengue in the United States Virgin Islands and cases imported to the continental United States of America 1977. In:

Dengue in the Caribbean 1977; Proceedings of a Workshop on Dengue in the Caribbean; 1978 May 8-11; Jamaica: Pan American Health Organization, 1979:75-82.

White PC, Moses EM, White ME. Influenza in Arkansas 1976-77. J Ark Ed Soc. 1978;5:188-192.

I edited the Arkansas Communicable Disease Bulletin in 1977 and the Saint Louis Encephalitis Surveillance Bulletin, issued by the Center for Disease Control, 1977-78.

I reviewed papers for:

Lancet
New England Journal of Medicine
Journal of Infectious Diseases
Epidemiology and Infection
Bulletin of the World Health Organization
Academic Medicine
The Health Research Board of Ireland